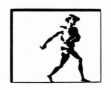

HELPING YOUR CHILD GROW SLIM

Safe Dieting for Overweight Children and Adolescents

Warren P. Silberstein, M.D.

AND

Lawrence Galton

SIMON AND SCHUSTER
NEW YORK

Published by Simon and Schuster
A Division of Gulf & Western Corporation
Simon & Schuster Building
Rockefeller Center
1230 Avenue of the Americas
New York, New York 10020
SIMON AND SCHUSTER and colophon
are trademarks of Simon & Schuster
Designed by Edith Fowler
Manufactured in the United States of America

10   9   8   7   6   5   4   3   2   1

Library of Congress Cataloging in Publication Data

Silberstein, Warren P.
  Helping your child grow slim
  Includes index.
  1. Obesity in children.   2. Reducing diets.
  3. Children—Nutrition.   4. Youth—Nutrition.
  I. Galton, Lawrence.   II. Title.
  RJ399.C6S56   613.2'5'088054   82-832
  ISBN 0-671-44280-5   AACR2

HELPING YOUR CHILD GROW SLIM

Safe Dieting for Overweight Children and Adolescents

Warren P. Silberstein, M.D.

AND

Lawrence Galton

SIMON AND SCHUSTER
NEW YORK

Library of Congress Cataloging in Publication Data

Silberstein, Warren P.
    Helping your child grow slim

    Includes index.
    1. Obesity in children.   2. Reducing diets.
3. Children—Nutrition.   4. Youth—Nutrition.
I. Galton, Lawrence.   II. Title.
RJ399.C6S56   613.2'5'088054   82-832
ISBN 0-671-44280-5   AACR2

To all children
who have ever been called "Fatso"

Contents

1
Why a Diet Guide
Unique for Children

Children are not simply little adults.

One of the great challenges for parents—and for pediatricians, too—is that children are constantly changing.

Childhood and adolescence are times of great growth—physical, mental, and emotional. And this growth is the foundation upon which later adult life will be built.

Is a child overweight?

Never should that problem be handled in the same fashion as it might be handled in adults.

For children and adolescents, a weight-control plan must do two things.

First, it must provide adequate nourishment for growth and development. Even an overweight child has nutritional needs for growth which must be met. The building blocks for growth include even some essential fats which the body cannot produce for itself.

Let a diet be severely restricted or unbalanced and it can be extremely dangerous for a child. During periods of malnourishment, children, however overweight, may experience significant harmful effects—among them decreased attention span, interference with learning, impaired ability to handle stress, and decreased capacity for fighting off infection.

Second, the plan must provide a diet with which the child can live comfortably. It must not seem *punitive*. And it should

9

teach the child a style of eating that can keep him trim and healthy for the rest of his life.

There is still another vital aspect to weight control in a child or adolescent that does not apply to adult dieters. An overweight adult who may have to lose 20 pounds knows that whether it takes 1 month or many months or a year or more, his goal is to reach an ideal weight that is 20 pounds below his present weight.

But a growing child who is 20 pounds overweight certainly should not be put on a diet to lose 20 pounds *because his ideal weight is constantly increasing as he grows.* So it is essential to set goals for the child dieter that are suitable for a growing youngster, not a growth-stable adult.

It is the purpose of this book to show you how to establish those goals for the *individual* child; how to determine what they should be considering both the child's weight and his growth pattern, and how then to design a diet for that child which you can be certain will be nutritionally sound and effective, and all the more so because it will be adaptable to his or her own food preferences and life-style.

I am addressing this book to parents—and to older children as well.

And I would urge parents to pass on to a younger child as much as possible of the information that follows.

May I add, too, that I write this book on the basis of experience not only as a pediatrician who has seen and treated a goodly number of overweight youngsters and come to know the special problems of their parents, but also as a formerly fat child myself.

W. P. S.

2
Setting Proper Goals

The child is overweight—by 10 pounds, 20, 25, or even more.
It's no rare condition.

Obesity, which has been called the number one public-health problem in the country, affects not only as many as 40 percent of adult Americans, according to some estimates, but also many hundreds of thousands of American children as well.

Exact figures for overweight incidence in children are hard to come by. The lowest estimates run to 10 to 13 percent of the child population—and that would be enough to represent a huge number. But many other estimates go much higher—to 30 percent and even more. According to a recent ten-state medical study which confined itself to children in the 11-to-18-year range, 39 percent of boys and 33 percent of girls are overweight.

And far from thinning out spontaneously, 80 percent of these overweight youngsters, unless something is done, become overweight adults.

So it might seem, at first blush, that any overweight child, like any overweight adult, would do well to slim down, to begin to lose pounds without delay.

But is that true? And if so, how many pounds how fast?

Remember, as we've noted, that for healthy growth a child must have adequate nutrition. At different ages, children have varying growth rates—but growth goes on. In early adolescence there is usually a very marked spurt of growth. During that spurt, some adolescents may grow as much as 6 inches in a year.

Complicated problem? Not really.

The answer to the seemingly complex question of how much weight a child should lose at any given point in his or her life is surprisingly simple. *In most instances, unless a child is extraordinarily obese, he or she shouldn't lose any weight at all!*

At this point, some charming young ladies, eager to fit into a special outfit by next month or even next week, may be somewhat disappointed. (Of course, there are times when a child or adolescent will want to set a specific goal for a weight loss of some number of pounds, and I assure you the advice in this book can help you achieve that while keeping you on a nutritionally sound diet.)

But many other young dieters-to-be will breathe a big sigh of relief at the thought of not having to lose weight.

That sigh of relief can be especially important when it comes from a younger child whose parent is helping him diet. Because no parent can impose a diet successfully on an un-cooperative child.

No less important, overzealous dieting to lose weight commonly fails in children.

It isn't only, as we've already noted, that diets aimed at large weight losses, even when well balanced, may not provide adequate nutrients for a child's growth.

In addition, the frustration produced by restrictive diets often leads to a child's breaking them and sometimes going on eating binges, with resultant weight gain.

Finally, restrictive reducing diets directed at producing quick and large weight losses do not teach the dieter healthy eating habits he or she can live with and depend upon for the rest of his or her life.

If you've ever dieted, you know that while half the battle may be staying on a diet, the other half is maintaining the weight loss. Only by learning proper eating habits can you avoid having to go on and off diets repeatedly, with weight bouncing up and down.

A SAFE, EFFECTIVE GOAL:
GROWING INTO THE RIGHT WEIGHT

A goal of zero weight loss—and at the same time, minimal or no weight gain—is a happy one for most children. It can be achieved on a nutritious diet without a great deal of suffering.

Even such a modest goal may require a marked change in eating habits as the dieter aims at not gaining any weight over an extended period of time, usually several years, until he or she grows into ideal weight.

With such a program, there can be healthy growth and development of the lean body mass while fat deposits decrease.

To understand how this would work, let's look at growth charts and then consider as an example the case of an overweight 7-year-old boy.

THE GROWTH CHARTS

They may seem complex at first glance, but they aren't really. Nor is the percentile concept. And you will want to— and readily can—understand both, since you will apply them to your own child.

The charts here are for boys. Later, in the Appendices, charts are provided for both boys and girls so that you can use those suitable for your child. We've added marks on these charts for the boy in our example, and we'll discuss those shortly.

As you see, there is one chart for stature or height, and a second chart for weight. Height is indicated in inches and weight in pounds along the vertical axes at the left of the respective charts, and in both cases age is indicated in years along the horizontal axes at bottom.

Each chart has a set of curves—and at the right, at the end of each curve, you find a number indicating a percentile. The percentiles shown are the 5th, 10th, 25th, 50th, 75th, 90th, and 95th.

The curves are based on data obtained from studies of

heights and weights of large numbers of children at various ages. And the percentiles show the distribution of heights and weights among those children and very probably, because the sampled children are representative, among all children.

And so, if a child is, for example, in the 50th percentile for height at his age, it means that half of all children his age are taller than he is and half of the same age are shorter.

If he is in the 10th percentile for height, that means that 90 percent of children his age are taller and 10 percent are shorter.

Similarly, for weight: If a child is in, say, the 40th percentile for weight at his age, 60 percent of children of the same age weigh more and 40 percent weigh less than he does.

The range of normal is broad. Many children cluster between the 25th and 75th percentiles. Others are in lower and higher percentiles. A child may be in the 90th percentile for height, for example, thus being considerably taller than a friend of the same age in the 10th percentile. But both are in the normal range.

It is only when a child is below the 5th percentile or above the 95th percentile that he may be considered unusual—out of the normal, everyday range. But that doesn't mean necessarily that an abnormal cause is involved. He could be healthy and his very tall or very short stature may be a matter of genes.

As for whether a child is of normal weight or is overweight, that is a matter of whether his height and weight percentiles are much the same or different.

For example, a child who is above the 95th percentile for both height and weight is not overweight. He is just big.

On the other hand, when a child is in a low percentile for height—perhaps 5th, 10th, or 25th—but in a higher percentile for weight, he is probably overweight even if he should be in the 50th percentile for weight, which would be average for his age.

Later you will be able to determine the height and weight percentiles for your child, and by comparing them, you will be able to establish what his ideal weight should be based on the percentile for height.

14

AN EXAMPLE

Now we can see how all this works out in the case of a 7-year-old boy who is 49 inches tall and weighs 74 pounds.

On the Stature for Age chart (page 16), you can run a finger up the left-hand side to the 49-inch height line, then follow that line across to the right to the age-7 vertical line. And where both lines intersect, you find an "x." As you see, this child is on the 75th-percentile curve for height.

Now, on the Weight for Age chart (page 17), run a finger up the left-hand side to the 74-pound line and follow that line across to the age-7 vertical line, where you find another "x." As you see, this youngster is above the 95th percentile for weight.

If he continues to grow in height and gain in weight at his usual rate, he will remain in the same percentiles. When he is 9½ years old, therefore, he will be 54½ inches tall and will weigh 100 pounds, as indicated by the "o" marks on the charts.

Now suppose instead that the child does not gain any weight over the next 2½ years. His weight at 9½ years will still be 74 pounds (indicated on the chart by a "+"). At that age, 74 pounds is in the 75th percentile—and since his height follows the 75th-percentile curve, 74 pounds, also in the 75th percentile, is his ideal weight.

What will the boy need to do to keep at 74 pounds over the next 2½ years?

To maintain any given weight and activity level, a certain number of calories are required. If consumption exceeds that number, pounds are added until the weight that will be maintained by the caloric intake is reached. If fewer calories are consumed than are burned up, pounds are lost until weight that will be maintained by the caloric intake is reached.

Our 7-year-old, assuming he is not unusually active or unusually sedentary, can maintain his 74 pounds for the next 2½ years on an intake of 32 to 36 calories for each of his 74 pounds as shown in the table in Appendix C, or a total of about 2,500 calories per day.

Now, of course, he could lose weight rather than maintain weight by consuming only 1,000 calories a day, or perhaps

BOYS FROM 2 TO 18 YEARS

STATURE FOR AGE

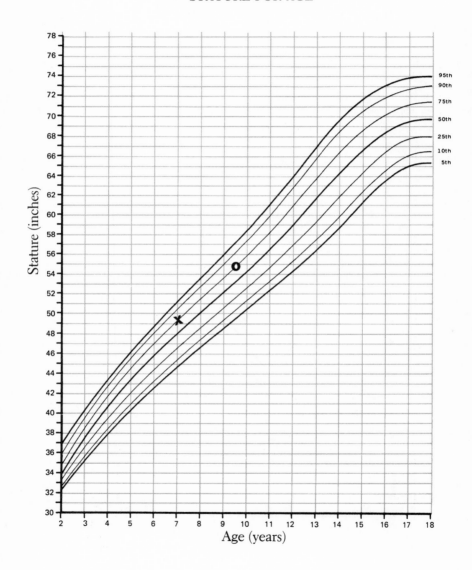

BOYS FROM 2 TO 18 YEARS
WEIGHT FOR AGE

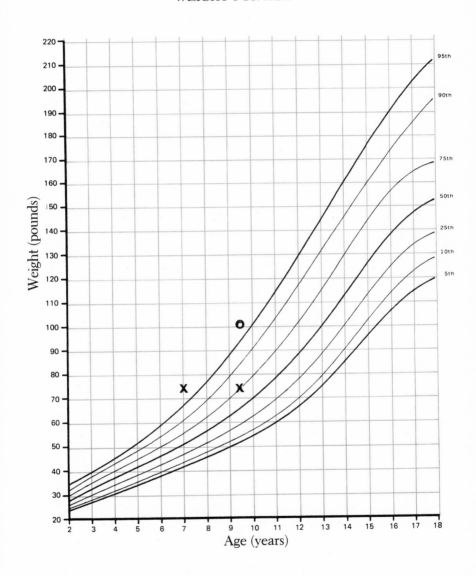

1,500—and the loss would be relatively fast. But it could be dangerous; he might well be nutritionally shortchanged.

Happily, on 2,500 calories a day there is no danger of nutritional impoverishment. For in fact, 2,500 calories a day meet the average daily requirements, as shown in Appendix C, of boys in the 10-to-12 age range.

LOSING WEIGHT

For children who are extraordinarily overweight and who would still be overweight even if they maintained their present weight for several years, zero weight gain would still be an improvement.

A reasonable goal, however, would be to aim for reducing to what the ideal weight can be expected to be 2 to 3 or 4 years into the future, based on the percentile curves.

Say, for example, that we have a 9-year-old who weighs 150 pounds. He is a big child—not uncommon for an obese youngster. At 55 inches, he is in the 90th percentile for height.

Now, with a weight of 150 pounds at age 9, even if he were to gain nothing at all, he would still be significantly above the 95th percentile for weight by the time he reaches age 13.

So in his case, reducing would be a good idea. The question is: How much should he lose—and over how long a period?

We have to take into account several important considerations.

For one thing, the diet must not be too restrictive for adequate growth, since the chances are that it will take several years to accomplish the proper weight loss. He may even begin to go through some of the changes of puberty—an added reason for not taking a chance on his not getting adequate nutrition.

Another reason it could take a long time is that for him to have become so obese, his eating habits, quite obviously, are far out of line. If we were to put him on a restrictive, quick-loss diet, he would have no chance to learn healthy new habits which would permit him to be eating normally when his weight is where it should be. For that, he needs to lose weight slowly.

And finally, this is a 9-year-old youngster who will almost

certainly give battle if the diet is too restrictive. Mother will have to enforce the diet; and once Mother becomes the enforcer, despite the best will in the world there will be adversary positions—and the more Mother tries to enforce the diet, the more against it the child will become.

So the diet has to be reasonably palatable, acceptable, satisfying. The child, of course, will have to change some of his eating habits. But I am convinced that no matter how overweight a youngster is, and no matter how much he may desire, say, ice cream and cake, if you give him a diet that does not leave him hungry, he can learn new eating habits and not eat ice cream and cake all the time but just once in a while.

We can set 130 pounds as his weight goal to be reached by age 13. Since he is in the 90th percentile for height, 130 pounds would place him in the 90th percentile for weight and be his ideal weight at 13.

How do we achieve the relatively modest weight loss of 20 pounds over a period of several years?

We can consult the table of "Average daily caloric requirements by age" in Appendix C. For our 9-year-old, that requirement is about 2,200 calories. We can be sure, given his obesity, that he is currently eating much more than that.

If he cuts down to between 2,200 calories and 2,700, which is the average requirement for a 13-year-old boy, he is going to lose weight—and he is going to lose it slowly, healthily.

We know that an average adult can be comfortable on 2,000 calories a day, and this youngster, on 2,200 to 2,700, is not going to starve and the diet is not going to be unbearable.

He will lose weight because he will be consuming fewer calories than his body needs to maintain his obese weight, even though his diet is not a reducing diet for a child his age. And because he will be getting the average number of calories required by a child his age, there is no way, if the diet is nutritious, for him to run into any problems with it.

THE OVERWEIGHT LATE-ADOLESCENT

Those adolescents who are overweight as they near the end of their growth period will need to reduce, aiming at their ideal weight for their predicted final height.

The predicted final height can be determined from the growth curves in Appendix A and/or the "Parent Mid-Stature Chart" in Appendix B, which makes use of parental heights. Final height is usually reached at about 18 years of age, but may occur earlier if there is early completion of sexual maturation.

To lose weight, then, find your ideal weight for height on the growth chart. To do this, note the predicted height at age 18 and the percentile in which it falls. Go on to note what the chart indicates for weight in the same percentile; this is your ideal weight.

You can then design your diet on the basis of your caloric requirements to maintain the ideal weight. (We will be discussing caloric requirements in more detail later.)

The end result of eating the caloric requirements for your ideal weight will be that when you reach your ideal weight your diet will be correct for maintaining that weight. And since the diet contains the proper number of calories for an average person of your age and height, if the diet is balanced (and more about that later), you cannot be nutritionally shortchanged.

ADJUSTMENTS

Since children are growing continuously, it is necessary to periodically adjust goals.

The method I have outlined here is, I firmly believe, the safest way for a growing child to lose weight. And since it is not aimed at producing rapid loss, and growth will continue during the loss period, the child's ideal weight and therefore caloric requirements will require upward adjustment.

Whether you choose to maintain zero weight gain or to lose weight, if you are still growing when you reach your ideal weight you will need to increase your food intake accordingly.

For many readers who choose to maintain zero weight gain and some who choose to lose weight, the suggestions in Chapters 6 and 7 and your bathroom scale will be all you need.

If you need a more formalized diet, you will know your caloric requirements and can choose between counting calories and using the exchange lists in Chapter 8.

3
How Diets Work

First, let me say that calories *do* count—and even if you, as a dieter, don't count calories, if you follow a diet and lose weight, it's by consuming fewer calories than you burn.

Second, there is no such thing as an easy diet. If a diet is well designed, it should provide a variety of foods you can enjoy and you shouldn't have to be hungry—but you do have to change your style of eating, and that takes work.

Finally, anyone who goes on a diet to lose weight with the idea that he will reward himself at the end by returning to his old eating habits is wasting his time. He will need to diet again in short order. And after having his weight go up and down on multiple diets, he will finally give up—discouraged, depressed, and still fat.

Anyone who is serious about dieting must make up his mind to change his eating habits for life. He has to find a diet he can live with and stay on permanently. Now, obviously—you know it well—if you're going to stay on a diet permanently, it has to be safe and nutritious; and if you start it in childhood, it has to be adequate to grow on.

The problem with many popular rapid-weight-loss diets is that they may not be at all sound to grow and develop on.

On the other hand, even though zero weight loss is less dramatic and may seem less immediately rewarding, as you learn the proper balance of foods to fill up on and get satisfaction from, and then eat other foods only as treats, you will grow up eating all foods in the right amounts, stay trim, and not even feel like a dieter.

Let us now examine what actually makes diets, including the rapid-weight-loss diets, work. In a later chapter we will look at some basics of nutrition. Following that, we will use our understanding of what makes diets work to devise some tricks for dieting. Then we can synthesize the information to make a sound slimming diet for a growing youth.

THE HALLMARKS

Diets, of course, range all the way from eating anything and everything you wish but counting the number of bites you take to eating only a single food such as grapefruit or cottage cheese for days on end.

But all have one thing in common: restriction. Either there is one thing or many things you cannot eat, or the quantities of some things are limited, or the quantity of everything is limited. The result, in each case, is a reduction in calories consumed.

All diets work to some extent by making you think before you eat. Particularly when you first start a diet, you can't just open the refrigerator and take out anything to eat. You have to think about what you can eat if you want to stay on the diet. In contrast, many overweight people are habituated to eating in response to stress or boredom. They grab whatever is handy to eat without even thinking about it. And very quickly thereafter, they are looking for something more to eat, because when you eat without thinking about it you are always left with an ill-defined sense of not being satisfied.

The method of cutting calories that is easiest to understand is calorie counting. For this, it's necessary to measure food by volume or weight and determine the caloric content by reference to a calorie table or book.

A change of 10 calories a day in either direction means a pound gained or lost in a year. That may not sound like very much; but the average 20-year-old, for example, who consumes 10 calories more than he burns every day will be 30 pounds overweight by the time he is 50.

An overweight child who is gaining at a rate of 10 pounds a

year and wants to stop gaining and keep his weight stable must cut down by 100 calories a day—the equivalent of 1 soft drink or 1 or 2 cookies.

Once ideal weight has been determined and, along with it, the caloric intake required daily to arrive at and maintain that weight, the way to reach the goal is by considering calories and not consuming more than the allowed amount.

VARIETIES OF DIETS

There is an almost endless stream of quick-loss diets, including the bizarre.

Some put the emphasis on foods that supposedly, because of enzymes in them, burn up more calories than they contain. Most often, grapefruit is called for, with eggs included for the sake of nutrition. Some years ago a U.S. Senate committee hearing on fad diets turned up fifty-one grapefruit-and-eggs diets. Often, these diets are offered under the name "Mayo" regimens, and the Mayo Clinic, a medical center of great repute, is kept busy denying, without qualification, that there is any connection.

Many popular diets are low in carbohydrates; some attempt to eliminate carbohydrates completely. It is a fact that many snack foods are largely made up of carbohydrates—and for many of us given to snacking, reduction or elimination of snack intake can be helpful in calorie restriction.

Diets very low in or without any carbohydrates can produce rapid initial weight loss for this reason: The body stores some carbohydrates in the form of glycogen, and the stored glycogen is hydrated, which means it contains water. With inadequate carbohydrates coming in from the diet, glycogen is mustered from the tissues and in the process its water is lost, producing quick weight loss. But the water—and weight—will be regained later, once dieting stops, as new stores of glycogen are deposited in the tissues.

Unfortunately, too, a diet very low in or without carbohydrates is almost always high in fat, and marked, unhealthy elevations of blood fats—which may be involved in artery disease—may occur in these circumstances.

23

Some diets are very low in fat. Fats are a concentrated source of calories, providing 9 calories per gram, in contrast to the 4 calories per gram for protein and carbohydrates. As a result, if you reduce the amount of fat in your diet, even if you replace it with an equal weight of carbohydrates or protein, you will cut calories. But very-low-fat diets can be difficult to stick with—for fats aid satiety.

Many diets provide complete weekly menus of low-calorie foods. For those easily tempted by high-calorie dishes, such diets, as long as they are followed, provide good control. Although you have to give some thought to what you are eating in order to follow the menus, you have no decisions to make about what to eat. Nothing is left to chance, and if you follow the menus to the letter, you're likely to lose weight. Of course, where amounts are specified, you must also measure out the correct quantities of food.

What is it that makes some foods low in calories?

Of course, lower fat content helps, since gram for gram, fat has more than twice as many calories as protein or carbohydrates, as we have noted.

But the lowest-calorie foods tend to be those high in fiber. Fiber is essentially indigestible and so can provide satisfying, stomach-filling bulk without adding calories.

Foods high in fiber include cereals such as old-fashioned, slow-cooking (not instant) oatmeal; shredded wheat; cereals labeled as being all-bran or largely made up of bran. Also: breads, muffins, and the like made with whole-meal flour (whole wheat or whole rye). And vegetables and fruits such as carrots, apples, brussels sprouts, eggplant, spring cabbage, corn, oranges, pears, green beans, lettuce, winter cabbage, peas, onions, celery, cucumbers, broad beans, tomatoes, cauliflower, bananas, rhubarb, potatoes, turnips, and seed-filled berries such as raspberries and blackberries.

On the other hand, highly refined carbohydrates—such as white flour and many cereals—provide very little fiber; it has been ground out. Refined sugar has practically no fiber at all.

Think about it: A slice of bread and 4 teaspoons of sugar have about the same number of calories. They are both carbohydrates. But which is more satisfying?

Essentially, sugar is a high-calorie flavoring. It does little to satisfy hunger. Another problem with refined sugar is that it is the prime cause of carbohydrate addiction.

Carbohydrate addiction—particularly sugar addiction—is perhaps the most prevalent and difficult-to-deal-with overeating habit in the United States. In our society, we are taught from early on that sweets are treats. We crave cake and cookies. What child would prefer to have a raw vegetable or piece of fresh fruit for a snack or dessert when a cookie is available? For that matter, who told kids that every time they eat their dinner they will get dessert? We did—when they were 2 years old and had the typical drop in appetite and loss of baby fat that most 2-year-olds experience.

The problem with sugar, which is in most of our treats, is that it is rapidly absorbed and causes a quick rise in sugar in the blood. This is followed by a rise in the insulin output from the pancreas to lower the level of sugar in the blood.

But insulin not only lowers blood sugar; it also increases the production of fat in fat cells.

And in addition, in many individuals who are particularly sensitive to sugar, within two hours the insulin will push the blood-sugar level far down, sometimes even lower than it was originally, leaving the sugar addict once again craving sweets.

Some children develop hypoglycemia (low blood sugar) after a highly sugared meal—and the hypoglycemia results in restlessness, decreased attention span, irritability, and fatigue. Refined sugars also play a major role in promoting tooth decay.

Those of us who have the misfortune to be addicted to drugs, caffeine, cigarettes, alcohol, gambling, or virtually anything other than food—and who manage to find the inner strength to quit—can avoid the temptation to resume addiction by complete avoidance.

It's another matter for those of us who have the misfortune to have an emotional, if not physical, dependence on eating. Should we decide to cut down, we cannot avoid temptation by avoiding food altogether.

The rigidity of some diets is sufficient for some to avoid tempting forbidden foods. And there are still others who actually go to the extreme of avoiding anything that reminds them of eating, relying instead on liquid protein diets.

But liquid protein diets have recently come under attack as being unsafe. They have been associated with a number of serious side effects, including irregular heart rhythms, fainting, muscular weakness, cramps, dry skin, and hair loss. A number of deaths have been reported after use of liquid protein diets.

The ultimate in food avoidance is the fast. For some people, the most difficult part of dieting is to get started. A 2-to-3-day fast may help to get the ball rolling.

After several days without eating, the dieter usually loses his craving for food. This result is not only psychological but also physical. After 2 to 3 days of fasting, the body's carbohydrate stores are depleted and the body burns fat.

And the breakdown products of fat, called ketone bodies, cause a loss of appetite. The presence of ketone bodies in the blood is called ketosis.

Several popular diets take advantage of the appetite-suppressant effect of ketosis, as we'll see. And in fact, ketosis can occur with almost any quick-loss diet.

Because it is not without hazard, ketosis deserves consideration here.

A SPECIAL WORD ABOUT KETOSIS DANGER

Ketosis is the result of incomplete burning of fat, which in turn is the result of inadequate carbohydrate intake—because of fasting, or a diet deliberately made very low in carbohydrates, or a diet very low in calories and therefore, incidentally, in carbohydrates.

Carbohydrates are the body's prime source of quick energy. And when carbohydrates are unavailable or in inadequate supply for energy, the body draws on its fat. The carbohydrate deficiency triggers hormonal activity and greatly increases the withdrawal of fat from fatty tissues. Large quantities of fat must then be handled—in chemical terms, they must be *oxidized*—and the quantities are more than the body cells can handle. So the handling—the oxidation—is incomplete, and ketones accumulate.

Ordinarily, ketones, when formed in small amounts, are eliminated readily from the body through exhalation via the lungs or through urine via the kidneys. But if large amounts of fat are burned incompletely, ketones can build up in the bloodstream faster than they can be eliminated.

If you and I go on a diet and lose weight slowly, we don't become ketotic. When we lose half a pound or a pound a week, the amount of fat burned produces no more ketone bodies than can be eliminated as rapidly as they are formed.

On the other hand, if we go on a quick-loss diet designed to get us burning up fat quickly enough to lose 10 or 20 pounds in a matter of a few weeks, we are going to have a ketone buildup. And that, I must point out, holds true even if the main source of your caloric intake is carbohydrate. Because it doesn't matter what you are eating; you are living on animal fat—your own—burning it up too rapidly for ketone elimination to keep pace with ketone production.

With ketosis, some people may have no overt problems. But we know that ketosis is an abnormal, unphysiologic state. Often there is a sweet or "fruity" odor to the breath—produced by acetone, a ketone body that is very volatile and is blown off in small amounts with air expired from the lungs.

Appetite loss may occur. Sometimes nausea and vomiting develop, blood fat becomes elevated, and ketosis on occasion can contribute to fatty liver and obstruction in the lymphatic system.

In my experience with children, if they become ketotic they may also become relatively hypoglycemic. On a diet low enough in calories to make them ketotic, they do not get an adequate source of quick energy. They may become restless and lose the ability to concentrate—and since most of our children spend a significant portion of the year in school, I think that is a big price to pay to lose weight.

CURRENTLY POPULAR DIETS

I mentioned earlier that several popular diets take advantage of the appetite-suppressant effect of ketosis. Many, many scores of diets appear in newspapers, magazines, and books, and we have no room in this book to review a large number of them. But I would like to comment briefly on the Scarsdale and Atkins diets.

27

The Scarsdale diet is said to result in weight losses of up to 20 pounds in 14 days.

Almost all carbohydrates and significant amounts of fat are banned. Only lean meats are allowed. All foods must be prepared without butter, all salads without oil or mayonnaise. No substitutions and no between-meal snacks are permitted, except for raw carrots and celery.

If an adult follows the highly restrictive Scarsdale diet, it provides about 1,000 calories a day. Within two days, there will usually be sufficient ketosis to reduce the appetite. No one is supposed to stay on the diet for more than 14 days at a time.

The Scarsdale diet has been criticized because it is unbalanced, too high in protein. Being low in calories, it induces weight loss. But being unbalanced, it is not a diet to be lived with permanently, and rapid weight gain is likely to occur as the dieter goes back to old eating patterns.

Certainly, I cannot recommend the Scarsdale diet because it significantly restricts calories and induces ketosis. It also does not take into account the varying needs of children of different sizes and ages.

The Atkins diet is one more version of the high-fat type of diet. Even more than a century ago, in 1864, William Banting, coffin maker to the Duke of Wellington, was advocating such a diet in his "Letter on Corpulence." It has had its periods of popularity ever since under varied names, including the Du Pont Diet which was fashionable in the early 1950s.

During the first week, the Atkins diet allows no carbohydrates—no fruit, vegetables, bread. But there is no limit on protein, fat, or calories. The dieter can load up on bacon and eggs, marbled steaks, and the like. In the second phase of the diet, small amounts of carbohydrates are gradually added.

Dr. Atkins has proposed a theory that because the body is burning only fat and not carbohydrates, calories are actually shed from the body in the form of ketone bodies. As a result, he says, you can consume more calories than you burn and still lose weight. In practice, I suspect that many of the people on this diet do not consume more calories than they burn because of the negative effect the ketosis has on their appetites.

The Atkins diet has been attacked by the Council on Foods and Nutrition of the American Medical Association as being a "bizarre regimen" and one "without scientific merit" and by *The Medical Letter,* a respected, independent rating publication going to physicians, as being "unbalanced, unsound and unsafe."

The Atkins diet has been criticized not only for the ketosis it induces but also because consumption of large amounts of saturated fats can elevate blood cholesterol levels and may contribute to coronary heart disease. Moreover, critics have pointed out, the very low carbohydrate intake can lead to fatigue, apathy, nausea, and heart irregularities; most of the weight lost with the very low carbohydrate intake is water and is quickly regained afterward; and certainly, this is not a diet with which one can live comfortably for the rest of his life.

When it comes to a child, even if there should be only the very smallest risk to health in a quick-loss diet, it seems unnecessary to take any risk at all if a child can become trim by learning good eating habits which allow him to enjoy all foods in reasonable amounts.

I don't think it wise for a child to commit himself to a lifetime of any kind of diet that severely restricts any kind of food. By now, I hope I have convinced you that successful dieting requires a lifetime commitment.

4
Health and
the Overweight Child

Not long ago, referring to adults, one physician wrote:

"If you're overweight, you're ill. And I mean seriously ill. Oh, that's not to say you won't get away with it for a long time. Or that you won't 'feel' perfectly well . . . But in the end, the fat will get you."

His reasons: "Carrying extra weight batters your arteries, plunders your heart, predisposes you to diabetes, and pounds away at the weight-bearing joints so that in the end a fat man wobbles where a thin man runs."

Children are destined to become adults, and any illness that affects adults because of obesity is of potential concern for the child who is overweight.

Coronary heart disease (with its resultant heart attacks), strokes, high blood pressure, adult-onset diabetes—these are illnesses that have a high association with overweight.

So have some other diseases as well.

The table below shows the principal causes of death among obese adults. Based on insurance-company statistics, it reveals the increased risks of being overweight in terms of the increased death rates from various diseases as compared with those of nonobese persons. For example, mortality from cardiovascular/renal (kidney) disease in obese men is 149 percent of normal; in obese women, it is 177 percent of normal. And mortality from diabetes in obese men is 383 percent of normal; in obese women, 372 percent of normal.

Principal Causes of Death Among the Obese

	MALE	FEMALE
Cardiovascular/renal disease	149%	177%
Stroke	159%	162%
Diabetes	383%	372%
Chronic kidney disease	191%	212%
Cancer of liver, gallbladder	168%	211%
Gallstones	152%	188%
Cirrhosis of liver	249%	147%
Appendicitis	223%	195%

Any child who is overweight and remains so into adulthood has that many more years of being overweight which could influence his propensity to be affected seriously by these illnesses.

Physicians now are finding high blood pressure as well as higher-than-normal levels of cholesterol and fats in the blood of a significant number of young children and adults—factors that may increase the risk of developing heart disease later in life.

The hazards in childhood

In addition to what the future may hold—the risks in adulthood if obesity is not conquered earlier—the fat child faces more immediate hazards than the child of normal weight.

Overweight children generally are more prone to respiratory disease, orthopedic problems, and accidents.

Because many are not eating the proper foods, they may also suffer subtler effects of poor nutrition—among them anemia, skin rashes, irritability, decreased attention span, and cravings for sugar.

There can be significant effects—many effects—on the musculoskeletal system.

In obese children fat tends to accumulate in the thighs, and many have great difficulty in walking without having their thighs rub together. Sores develop and make them uncomfortable.

31

Intertrigo is a rash that may develop when two moist folds of skin keep rubbing together. It can become very sore—and it can develop not only between the legs but almost anywhere —under the arms, between two folds of fat around the neck.

Because of the fat around the thighs, many obese youngsters tend to separate their legs in order to walk. That puts abnormal stress on the hips, and one possible result of that stress is a condition seen in some overweight adolescents, usually boys—slipped femoral capital epiphysis.

What happens is that the growth plate, the femoral capital epiphysis, which is at the end of the hipbone where the leg attaches to the hip, is subjected to an abnormal force which causes it to slide down off the end of the bone.

The onset is usually insidious. At first there may be some stiffness of the hip which improves with rest. A limp may follow, and then hip pain which radiates down the thigh to the knee. As the condition advances, there may be pain on motion of the affected hip and limitation of motion, along with knee pain, limp, and rotation of the affected leg. Surgical repair may be needed.

Some obese children become swaybacked because of the increased weight load from the abdomen. The spine becomes curved in an S-shape. The lower spine, with the belly hanging from it, tends to swing forward—and to compensate, the child has to pull his shoulders farther back, putting abnormal stress on the spine.

Meanwhile, the back muscles are trying to support extra weight on a spine that is no longer straight, so that the weight is not distributed straight down. Back problems may develop —with the pain and limited mobility or immobility reinforcing the sedentary life-style, which only goes to make for more obesity.

THE EMOTIONAL IMPACT

Perhaps the most difficult aspect of obesity for the child is its effect on his emotional and social development.

Even the overweight adult has difficulty dealing with the rejection and discrimination he faces as a result of obesity.

The child, whose self-image is still forming, may develop a crippling lack of self-esteem.

Other children will be much less subtle than adults in their rejection of a fat child. Taunting is common. Even adults will tend to consider an obese child to be less cute than other children and treat him differently.

There have been studies indicating that teachers may tend to grade a fat child lower than a thin child. Later, the fat young person may find himself or herself more likely to be excluded by sororities, fraternities, and other social organizations and even discriminated against by some colleges and still later by some employers.

Discrimination, once it starts, may reinforce a fat child's poor self-image and may even lead to a vicious cycle of overeating, increased loss of self-respect, and still more overeating.

Perhaps the worst rejection an overweight child may face is unintentional rejection by his mother. As the child becomes increasingly heavy, she may become unable to pick him up readily—at an early age when many children need and get such attention.

And if in her efforts to help her overweight child, the mother simply cuts down on food for him and cuts out treats, the child is likely to perceive this as yet another rejection.

Because weight and dieting are such potentially touchy subjects for the obese child, the emphasis must be placed on reeducation in eating habits and food preferences and not on cutting down. The goal of the diet must be reasonable so that the diet will not seem oppressive. And the child must be motivated so he can maintain a positive attitude about his diet. I believe the zero-weight-gain plan will meet with approval from most young critics, and this is another reason it is particularly suitable for children.

A PERSONAL "INSIDE LOOK"

It may be difficult for someone who was never a fat child to appreciate fully the travails obesity can entail in childhood.

I have no such difficulty. As I indicated earlier, I was a fatty.

It just so happens that although there is something of a familial propensity to have some degree of obesity in my family, when I was a young child neither my father nor my mother was overweight.

But neither made any extra-special effort to keep us kids— my twin brother and my sister as well as me—from overindulging, perhaps because they had no problem and in early childhood neither did we.

My mother cooked proper meals; we always had good food in the house. And we also had cookies when we wanted, and all the cake that seized our fancy at any given time.

Nobody paid much attention. I was, in fact, a skinny kid; my brother was too; and my sister wasn't overweight.

And then, about the time I was 5, my skinny parents suddenly found they didn't have two skinny twin boys anymore; we were turning into twin blobs. It happened relatively quickly, and none of us realized it was happening until it was a fact.

As a fat child, I was always among the last to be picked for a team. It's hard to decide whether I became fat because I was physically awkward or was physically awkward because I became fat. But by the time I got to school, I was no longer skinny.

I think that, universally, fat kids experience the same setbacks: rejection, not fitting in, knowing even before you are rejected that you don't fit in, not being able to live up to your potential.

I think that obesity greatly increases the struggles of a youngster during adolescence. The adolescent has a constantly changing body and becomes very self-conscious about whether his or her body is the way it is supposed to be. Starting out as a little boy or girl, he or she develops into an adult with fully mature sexual organs.

During the entire period of adolescence, young people have as one of their prime concerns whether or not their development is normal. Many times they become ashamed of their bodies during the changes because they don't know what is normal. And even the normal-weight adolescent may be too embarrassed to show his or her body to anyone and ask and so resolve any doubts. Obesity compounds that problem manyfold, because you start out knowing your body is *not* normal and you shrink from even the thought of undressing in front of a physician or anyone else.

In one way, I was a relatively fortunate fatty.

I went to school in the early years in New York City, and there were vast numbers of kids to a grade and many classes for a grade. I was able without great difficulty to find a reasonable number of peers who had some of my problems, and some of my interests as well.

But that was only a short-term advantage. Eventually we moved away from New York City, and I found myself in the fifth grade in a school system with only a small fraction of the City's enrollment.

Here, I was facing the real world—with kids who weren't overweight, who didn't think that books were the best things in the world, who wanted to play ball and climb monkey bars —and I was, obviously, an outsider.

It's true that kids can sometimes be cruel and make fun of almost anything—but they are usually much more willing to pick on other kids who are overweight than on kids who are skinny.

Fortunately, I had a twin brother pretty much like me but a bit more physically adept, and he was able to bridge the gap a little.

WHY CHILDREN BECOME OVERWEIGHT

Any discussion of health and obesity warrants considering what can cause the obesity.

The main point I wish to make here is that there are very few disease states capable of causing obesity, and that most obesity is not in fact the result of disease.

Nevertheless, since there is a possibility, though rare, that a disease may be contributing to excessive weight, before starting any diet a child should be evaluated by his doctor.

Generally, a complete physical examination is sufficient. But in some circumstances the physician may wish to check adrenal-gland function, thyroid function, blood sugar and salts, cholesterol, and triglycerides. Urinalysis and blood-pressure measurement are essential parts of the complete physical.

Hypothyroidism—thyroid-gland deficiency—is frequently blamed for obesity in adults. It may in fact be more common than we realize, because subtle thyroid-deficiency states cannot be recognized without testing for them.

Children respond differently to thyroid disease than do adults, because children are still growing. The main problem seen with thyroid deficiency in children is growth failure rather than obesity.

Some people have tried using thyroid hormone to bring about weight loss—but in studies in which thyroid hormone was used along with caloric restriction, weight loss was predominantly and undesirably of lean body mass rather than fat.

It's also worth noting here that hypothyroid patients often tend to show relatively little interest in eating. Many factors may contribute to this, but one reason indicated by recent studies is that food does not taste very good to many hypothyroid patients. A substantial number of them turn out to have defects of taste and smell, and they have difficulty in actually tasting sweet, sour, salty, and bitter foods and in smelling common food odors. Such defects are largely corrected when they are treated with thyroid hormones.

Cushing's syndrome, in which excessive amounts of hormones are produced by the adrenal glands, can cause obesity. But patients with this disorder have a round face, a heavy and protuberant abdomen, and peculiar distribution of fat over the shoulders, cheeks, and hips and should be readily recognizable by your doctor. Because it leads to a metabolic derangement, Cushing's also results in growth failure. Along with being identifiable, it is treatable.

Some relatively rare neurologic disorders can cause obesity, but they also produce other symptoms which would lead a physician to correct diagnosis. For example, very uncommon brain tumors can be responsible for excessive weight gain, but they also cause other symptoms—such as lack of balance, slurring of speech, vomiting, vision disturbances—which help point to them.

Even when a glandular disturbance or other physical disease is not involved, there is evidence to indicate that over-weight people cannot eat as many calories as their lean counterparts without gaining weight. Decreased levels of physical activity, lower excretion of calorie-rich materials have all been postulated as reasons.

The point to be made is that whether your problem is a genetic predisposition to be fat, or a low metabolic rate, or even a glandular condition, you cannot gain weight unless you consume more calories than you burn.

If you want to be slim, there is no point in crying that it's not fair your friends can eat more than you can. Actually, you can eat as much as your friends once you learn which foods you can eat a lot of to fill up on, and which foods you must take in limited portions.

5
Basic Nutrition

Vitamins are essential to good nutrition; but they are not the essence of good nutrition.

The American public has been greatly misled as to what vitamins can do. In the face of a poorly balanced diet, a vitamin pill, no matter how potent, waves no magic wand to provide needed balance.

For a growing child, a most essential nutrient is protein. In addition, fat plays a vital role in the body, and although the overweight child may need a low-fat diet, he will still require some fat in order to obtain the small amount of essential fatty acids the body does not produce. He will require some fat, too, in order to be able to absorb fat-soluble vitamins.

Certainly no one food should be singled out as a villain in the battle of the bulge. As a fat little child, I often asked my mother, "Is this fattening?" She always replied, "If you eat enough of anything, it's fattening." She was right. On the other hand, if we eat the right amounts of everything, we should be healthy, satisfied, and not overweight.

WHAT A CHILD'S BODY NEEDS

The human body, obviously, is complex. It's to be expected, then, that its nutritional needs would be complex. They are, in the sense that many nutrients are required, no one of which is predominant.

For health, the needs of both child and adult are much alike. But if anything, meeting those needs is even more critical in the growing child.

What's needed is a proper mix of protein, carbohydrate, fat, vitamins, and minerals—all in suitable proportions and coming from a variety of foods. The variety can help to make certain that other vital nutrients—still-unknown vitamins, minerals, and perhaps other nutrients—are provided.

PROTEIN

Although protein is a basic requirement, our society tends to greatly exaggerate the need for it.

The heart, the liver, the kidneys, brain tissue, muscles—all are composed mainly of protein. And in fact, an adequate protein supply is required by every body cell, since the cell wall is protein and so is as much as one-fifth of the total cell mass.

Proteins are the most complex of natural compounds. They are made up of small constituent units known as amino acids. As proteins are digested, they are broken down into their amino-acid units, and the body can then construct from them its own particular kinds of needed proteins—those which make up its enzymes, disease-fighting antibodies, hormones, blood, and other cells and tissues.

More than twenty different amino acids are found in proteins. The body itself can produce many. But there are some "essential" amino acids—so called because the body is unable to synthesize them. They are, therefore, dietary essentials and include lysine, valine, isoleucine, leucine, threonine, tryptophan, methionine, phenylalanine, and histidine.

Many foods contain protein. All flesh—from fish, fowl, cattle, and other mammals—is rich in it. Cow's milk has a high content—three times as much as human milk. Cheeses often have still more protein. Cereals contain about 5 to 10 percent by weight. Fruit contains a little—about 1 percent by weight. Vegetables, particularly peas and beans, have a greater proportion than fruit.

Protein foods containing large amounts of the essential

amino acids are known as complete proteins and include those from animal sources, such as meat, eggs, and milk.

Vegetable proteins are incomplete; that is, a single vegetable does not contain all essential amino acids. But all can be obtained from a mix of vegetables.

You can obtain complete protein, for example, by combining peanut butter and whole-wheat bread, rice and beans, nuts and beans, macaroni and cheese, and cereal and milk.

How much protein is necessary? Vital as it is, much less than many people think.

Research has shown that half a gram of protein for every kilogram (2.2 pounds) of body weight is more than adequate for normal maintenance in an adult, providing a good margin of safety.

For growing children and adolescents, the studies suggest a protein intake of 2 to 3 grams per kilogram of body weight.

Even at 3 grams per kilogram, a 100-pound youngster, for example, would require no more than about 135 grams, or 5 ounces, a day.

But Americans eat large amounts of protein—on the order of 90 to 100 grams a day for adults: well in excess of adult requirements. And youngsters generally consume more than they actually need.

Extra protein can contribute to obesity. A gram of protein has a caloric value of about 4—no less or more than a gram of carbohydrate.

Moreover, foods don't contain protein alone and nothing else. For example, in terms of calories, about 20 percent of a T-bone steak is protein and 75 percent is fat. Cheddar cheese is 25 percent protein and 75 percent fat. (It's worth noting here that ounce for ounce, chicken has more protein than steak, while steak has 1½ to 2½ times as many calories and 2 or more times as much fat, depending upon the cut of steak.)

There is virtually no such thing as fat-free meat. Certainly, meat eaten in the right quantities is good for us, but the over-emphasis on meat in our society tends to make us overeat meat, and that means we are putting away quantities of calories we don't need.

Some overweight people may prefer meat to all other food. But that is not necessarily true for most. Yet from early on in childhood, many have been told they should eat meat, lots of it. Parents, with the best of intentions, often insist on it.

Of course kids should eat meat. But adults should be well satisfied with a quarter-pound hamburger, and there is no health reason for a small child to be eating as much. Even for an older child, 2 to 3 ounces of meat at a meal is more than sufficient.

Keeping protein intake moderate will, at the same time, almost certainly moderate the intake of fat which so often goes along with protein. And that can mean a significant reduction in total calories, since fat contains more than twice as many calories as proteins or carbohydrates—9 calories per fat gram versus 4 for the others.

CARBOHYDRATES

Carbohydrates, which include all starches and sugars, have been misguidedly assigned a low prestige value among foods.

Supposed to be high in calories and low in nutritional values, they are neither.

On the contrary, carbohydrate-containing foods contain many vital nutrients and are our major sources of plant fiber, vitamin C, and the B vitamins—niacin, thiamine, and riboflavin—and many important trace elements as well.

Carbohydrates, ounce for ounce, are no more fattening than protein and have less than half the calories of fat.

If, for example, you eat a 5-ounce potato, without butter or sour cream, you consume 110 calories. In comparison, a 5-ounce steak provides 500 calories, since it has more fat than protein. Yet it's common to see weight watchers mistakenly leave potato unfinished on the plate while consuming every last bit of steak.

Carbohydrates include the many sugars. Among them are fructose, the sweetest, found in honey, ripe fruits, and many vegetables; lactose, a sugar in milk; maltose, a sugar from malt or digested starch; and sucrose, the table sugar obtained from sugarcane and beets and maple trees and sorghum.

Starches are made up of complex instead of simple sugars and are not sweet. Starches are found in tubers such as potatoes; in seeds such as peas, beans, peanuts, and almonds; and

41

in roots such as carrots and beets. Our biggest sources, however, are cereal grains—wheat, rye, rice, barley, corn, millet, and oats.

A major function of carbohydrates is to supply energy. Starches are absorbed from the intestinal tract only after they have been converted to glucose, the blood sugar. This takes place relatively quickly, and energy from carbohydrates is rapidly available and rapidly used.

Glucose is an essential nutrient and energy source for muscles and other organs, especially the brain. An inadequate supply for the brain and nervous system produces feelings of weakness, dizziness, nausea, and hunger.

In providing energy, carbohydrates spare protein so it can be used for its prime purposes of body building and repair.

The starchy foods we eat contribute more than caloric energy. Potatoes, for example, contain significant amounts of vitamin C and the B vitamin nicotinic acid, and whole-grain cereals contain many vitamins and protein as well.

Moreover, carbohydrates also help the body utilize other nutrients such as fiber, vitamins, and minerals.

Yet in recent years, carbohydrates have been undervalued and underused in the American diet.

Worldwide, through much of history, carbohydrates have been the major source of calories. And currently in much of the world carbohydrates still contribute 60 to 75 percent of total calories.

But in the United States carbohydrate consumption has declined from about 60 percent of total diet calories at the turn of the century to 46 percent now.

And the greatest decline has been in the nourishing complex carbohydrates, while intake of "empty" calories from sweetened food has increased.

Where in 1909, 1 pound of sugar was consumed for every 10 pounds of fruits, vegetables, and cereal products in the American diet, now we eat a pound of sugar for every 5 pounds of fruits, vegetables, and cereals. As a recent White Paper of the American Dietetic Association has pointed out, "We are not eating the starchy vegetables and cereals that provide a balance between complex and simple carbohydrate, and also provide vitamins, minerals, and fiber."

FATS

Fats serve many purposes in the body.

They are required in every body cell as essential constituents of cell membranes that regulate the cell's intake of nutrients and excretion of waste. Stored in layers under the skin as reserves, fats act as insulators, helping to maintain body temperature. They provide the body with essential fatty acids, and transport and help in the absorption of vital fat-soluble vitamins—A, D, E, and K. They help to maintain the health of the skin.

Fats provide an effective way to store energy. An ounce, or any other weight, of stored fat in the body will yield about 2¼ times as much energy as an equivalent weight of protein or carbohydrate.

Actually, a little under half the fat calories in the typical American diet come from visible sources such as butter and margarine (80 percent fat), oils and shortenings (100 percent fat), and bacon (50 percent fat).

More fat calories come from so-called invisible sources. The marbling in beef, for example, is not always obvious. Cream cheese and hard cheeses, deep-fried foods, creamed soups, chocolate, ice cream—all are rich in fat.

A large proportion of the calories in nuts, avocados, and oil-packed sardines, tuna, and salmon are fat calories. That's true as well for frankfurters, bologna, salami, gravies and sauces, pies, cookies, whipped toppings, and coffee whiteners.

You expect rich desserts to have a lot of sugar. Yet they often contain more fat than sugar.

On the other hand, in lean lamb and most fish, fat content is 8 percent or less; in milk and shellfish, 2 to 4 percent; in fruits, vegetables, and most bread, less than 1 percent.

Despite the fact that Americans are increasingly fat-conscious, many of us take in far more fat than we need. Toward the beginning of the century, fat made up 32 percent of the American diet; today, the figure is 42 percent.

That is a lot of fat—in terms of weight control and in terms, too, of the possible role of fats, particularly certain types, in heart disease.

Fatty acids and the fats they form are classified as saturated or unsaturated. Common unsaturated fatty acids are liquid at room temperature. By a process of hydrogenation—the addition of hydrogen—they can be made saturated and turned into solid fats. One example of such hydrogenation is margarine.

Studies suggest that unsaturated fats—also called polyunsaturated—may be less likely to be used harmfully by the body. It appears that the concentration of cholesterol in the blood may be increased by saturated fats, which mostly occur in animal foods, such as meat, butter and eggs. On the other hand, unsaturated fats, which occur in large amounts in vegetable oils such as corn and safflower oil, may help reduce the amount of cholesterol in the blood. And cholesterol is believed by some researchers to be a major factor in the artery disease leading to heart attacks.

VITAMINS

Actually, vitamins are not nutrients in themselves; rather, they act on nutrients. As part of body enzyme systems, they play vital roles in helping to regulate the rate at which chemical reactions take place.

They are essential for the release of energy, for the building of tissue, and for controlling the body's use of food. By themselves, they provide no energy and build no tissues.

The amounts required are very small—measured in milligrams, micrograms, and International Units. A milligram is one-thousandth of a gram; and it takes 28 grams to make an ounce. A microgram is only one-millionth of a gram. International Units, also tiny quantities, measure the potency, or ability to promote growth or cure a deficiency disease.

Most vitamins must be obtained from the diet. Only three known vitamins are made in the body. With sufficient exposure to sunlight, vitamin D is produced in the skin. Niacin, a B vitamin, can be synthesized by the body from the amino acid tryptophan. And vitamin K is made by bacteria normally present in the intestine.

Each vitamin serves a special function—and in some cases several functions—beyond the capacity of any other sub-

44

stance. And vitamin deficiencies are specific. In fact, part of the definition of a vitamin is that its lack leads to a specific set of deficiency symptoms which disappear when the vitamin is supplied.

Vitamins are classified by their solubility in fat or water. The fat-soluble vitamins—A, D, E, and K—are stored in the body. The water-soluble vitamins—C, thiamine, niacin, and others—are not stored to any significant extent.

Here are some of the major functions of individual vitamins:

Vitamin A: Helps to form and maintain the skin and also the mucous membranes which line the intestinal tract and such body openings as the nasal passages. Also acts in certain visual processes, forming visual purple and promoting adaptation in dim light.

Vitamin C (ascorbic acid): Forms cementing substances that hold cells together in tissues. Also strengthens blood vessels, aids in wound healing, increases resistance to infection, and helps in the body's utilization of the mineral iron.

Vitamin D: Helps the body absorb calcium from food and aids the incorporation of calcium and phosphorus into bone.

Vitamin E: Helps protect unsaturated fatty acids and vitamin A from destruction by oxygen.

Vitamin K: Aids blood clotting to avoid hemorrhaging.

Thiamine (B_1): Aids utilization of carbohydrate, promotes normal appetite, contributes to nervous-system functioning.

Riboflavin (B_2): Aids in cell energy production, promotes healthy eyes and skin.

Niacin (B_3): Promotes normal appetite, aids digestion, contributes to health of skin, nerves, digestive tract. Also participates in synthesis of fat, use of carbohydrate, and tissue respiration.

Pyridoxine (B_6): Helps regulate use of protein, fat, and carbohydrate, and aids in regeneration of red blood cells.

Folic acid (folacin): Contributes to blood formation and functioning of various enzyme and other body systems.

Vitamin B_{12} (cobalamin): Participates in blood formation and nerve-tissue maintenance.

Biotin: Helps regulate carbohydrate use and aids formation and use of fatty acids.

Panthothenic acid: Helps regulate use of carbohydrate, fat, and protein for energy production.

As we've noted, vitamin deficiencies produce specific symptoms.

For example, inadequate vitamin A can lead to night blindness, failure of bone growth, tooth decay. Vitamin C deficiency can cause skin roughness, hemorrhages, loosening of teeth, bleeding of gums. Lack of sufficient vitamin D may result in growth retardation, bowing of legs, malformation of teeth. Vitamin E deficiency can lead to breakdown of red blood cells.

And these are symptoms that can result from deficiencies of other vitamins: From insufficient vitamin K: hemorrhage; thiamine: leg cramps, muscle weakness, mental confusion; riboflavin: eye sensitivity to light, cracks at corners of mouth, skin disturbances about nose and lips; niacin: skin disorders, smooth tongue, mental confusion, irritability, diarrhea; pyridoxine: nausea, dizziness, anemia, kidney stones, skin disorders, smooth tongue; folic acid: anemia, smooth tongue, diarrhea; Vitamin B_{12}: pernicious anemia with appetite loss, abdominal pain, weight loss, tongue burning, irritability, depression.

All vitamin needs can usually be supplied by a well-balanced diet. For example, either a medium stalk (about 6 ounces) of broccoli, or half a cantaloupe, or half a cup of orange juice can meet the vitamin C need. For vitamin A, half a cup of peas and carrots or half a cup of spinach will suffice. Three ounces of liver (pork, calf, or beef) will furnish the riboflavin requirement, and two cups of milk (including low-fat or skim) will provide half the daily requirement. For niacin, three ounces of water-pack tuna or the same amount of chicken or turkey will provide half of what is needed.

MINERALS

Among the nutrients known to be essential to human health are more than a dozen minerals. They are required for muscle contraction, heartbeat control, nerve-impulse conduction, bone and teeth formation and maintenance.

Occurring in soil, minerals are taken in by plants, from which they are absorbed by animals, and we in turn get minerals from both plants and animals.

Some minerals are required in substantial amounts and are called macronutrients. They include calcium and phosphorus, which are required for bone and teeth formation, normal nervous-system functioning, and still other activities. Milk and dairy products are good sources of calcium, and phosphorus is available in many foods, including milk, peas, beef, pork, tuna, peanuts, cottage cheese.

Magnesium, another macronutrient, is involved in many aspects of body chemistry and in nerve and muscle activity. It is plentiful in seafood, meats, nuts, whole grains, and wheat bran, and occurs in moderate amounts in leafy green vegetables, fruits, and dairy foods.

The fourth macronutrient, potassium, has among its functions the transmission of nerve impulses and release of energy from carbohydrates, proteins, and fats. It is widely distributed in foods, especially in meats, milk, vegetables, and fruits—and oranges, tomatoes, and bananas are good sources.

Trace minerals—also known as micronutrients—are essential for health although needed only in tiny amounts.

Iodine, for example, is needed only in the amount of 150 micrograms (millionths of a gram) per day, yet is crucial to the functioning of the thyroid gland. Common sources include seafood and iodized salt.

Iron goes into the making of hemoglobin, the pigment in red blood cells that transports oxygen from lungs to all body tissues. Meats are good sources. And iron is also found in eggs, oysters, sardines, shrimp, green vegetables, dry beans, nuts, prunes, dates, and raisins.

Chromium, of which only 0.2 milligram per day is needed, helps insulin to act in the body's proper handling of the blood sugar, glucose. It occurs in meats and whole grains.

Copper, needed in amounts of only about 3 milligrams a day, plays a part in bone and muscle development and nervous-system activity. Good sources include shellfish, organ meats, nuts, legumes, and raisins.

Manganese, found in nuts, legumes, whole grains, and tea, is needed only in amounts of 5 milligrams a day, but is required for bone formation, nervous-system functioning, and reproduction.

Only one-half milligram of molybdenum is needed daily and can be obtained from cereals and legumes. It is required in some body enzyme systems and aids utilization of iron.

Selenium, which is believed to protect membranes and other fragile structures from oxygen damage, is found in grains and onions. Only 0.2 milligram per day suffices.

Zinc is needed for growth, for sexual maturation, and as a component of many enzymes. The requirement is 15 milligrams a day, and good sources include seafood, nuts, meat, eggs, and green leafy vegetables.

One important fact about minerals is that a balance of them is needed—and more is not better and can, in fact, be hazardous. For example, too much zinc intake may cause copper deficiency.

Unquestionably, the best and safest way to get the proper amounts of known essential minerals—and of other unknown as well as known vital nutrients—is through a balanced and varied diet.

And when you come to the Diet Exchange Lists in Chapter 8, you will find that they are simple, useful tools for helping to ensure balance and variety even as they serve other valuable purposes, including simplifying the consideration of calories and your own design of an effective, individualized weight-control program.

Even before the Lists, however, here in Chapters 6 and 7 are stratagems and principles that can go far to make the weight-control program successful.

6
Tricks of Dieting

The tricks of dieting are not tricks in the sense of being cheating devices. No matter what diet you are on, you must follow it if you expect to reach your goal. The tricks are aids for starting—and staying on—your diet.

They are stratagems to help make you aware of what you eat, where you eat, when you eat, and why you eat. Then, armed with that awareness, you can avoid or change those situations which provoke overeating and the eating of wrong foods.

There are also stratagems for changing, beneficially, the very way in which you eat.

And they include, as well, simple cutback and substitution maneuvers which can contribute significantly to effective weight control.

THE LOG

One of the first and most important things an overweight child can do—or a parent may need to do for the child—is keep a log of everything eaten.

Eating too much is very often a learned behavior. To some extent, almost all of us do some of our eating without really being hungry. But the obese—both children and adults—tend to be far ahead. Commonly, it appears, they do much of their eating not in response to internal hunger pangs but rather because of external cues—the time of day; the sight or smell of food. Frequently, they nibble without thinking while watching television or reading. Many eat simply because it is mealtime and even when not hungry may finish everything in front of them. Often, too, they tend to eat, without regard to hunger, when lonesome or bored or depressed.

A daily log—an inventory of eating and eating habits—can be most helpful.

The log should note everything that is eaten—the type and amount of food, where and when the eating takes place, the time spent eating, and any activity while eating.

It can be valuable, too, to include an indication of what stimulated the eating. Was it because of hunger? Or did, for example, a picture of food in a magazine or a commercial on TV induce the desire to eat?

Many who keep such logs are surprised to discover that they eat much more than they thought they did. Many also discover that keeping the log, and thus becoming more aware of their eating behavior, helps them in itself to control what they eat. They actually eat less when they keep a record of their eating.

And a log can be helpful, too, in pointing to specific eating-behavior habits which, if changed—often with relative ease—can contribute greatly to weight control.

A PRIME CHANGE

Eat slowly. For several reasons, this is of major importance.

Many overweight children tend to eat quite rapidly. Yet for one thing, eating slowly can allow time to enjoy food and to experience a greater sense of satisfaction even though fewer calories are consumed.

Slow eating also gives satiety a chance to work before over-eating can occur. Research indicates that it takes about 20 minutes after the start of a meal for the satiety center in the brain to get the signal that all is well and no more food is required: satiety has been reached.

So it can help greatly if an overweight child is encouraged to take his or her time, to spend at least 20 minutes at a meal —and if other family members who may not already be reasonably slow eaters help by slowing down.

Any one or several of a number of simple techniques can be used to help the child learn to moderate the eating pace. They include:

- Taking smaller bites.
- Chewing each bite longer, savoring and enjoying the taste.
- Laying fork or spoon down after each bite or after several bites and waiting until after swallowing before picking up the fork or spoon again.
- Taking a sip of water after every few bites.
- Counting bites and pausing, after every three or four, for a minute or so before taking another.
- Using a napkin more frequently.

OTHER IMPORTANT EATING-BEHAVIOR MODIFICATIONS

These are "rules" which are pertinent for many, even most, overweight children. An older child may be able to apply them for himself or herself. Patient parental guidance for a younger child will be very much worthwhile.

- Eat only at the table—and that applies not only for meals but for any and all snacking.
- Don't engage in other activities—especially reading or watching TV—while eating.
- Take only the portion you intend to eat to the table. Do not bring any platters, jars, boxes, bowls, or pots of food along.
- Be honest with yourself and don't take more than what you know to be a reasonable portion based on what your diet requires.
- Don't feel obliged to finish something on your plate when you have had enough.
- Don't take a second portion of anything except those vegetables in the unlimited list in the next chapter.
- Measure your portions if you are not sure how much you are eating.
- Use the lowest-calorie version of whatever food you intend to eat. Of course, avoid artificial ingredients. For dairy

51

foods, use low-fat and skim milk products. Choose thinly sliced bread.

• Drink a large glass of water before each meal.

• Fill up on plenty of low-calorie, high-fiber vegetables (listed in the next chapter) as part of your meal.

• Do not eat dessert at a meal if you are no longer hungry. Save it for when you need a snack.

• Eat three satisfying meals a day, unless you're not hungry at mealtime. Don't skip a meal for the sake of diet. Skipping meals usually makes it more difficult to stay on a diet.

• Reward yourself each weekend with one portion of a treat you have been avoiding all week; but don't overdo and lose ground.

OMISSION MANEUVERS:
THE SMALL ONES CAN COUNT HEAVILY

You may be surprised how much small omissions—not difficult at all to make—can contribute to effective weight control.

In fact, it's even possible that in some cases, a combination of several such omissions may be enough to achieve the control.

Consider:

If, for example, you omit just one pat of butter or margarine daily, you can avoid gaining 3½ pounds in the course of the next year.

Over that time period, too, the omission of a single slice of bread or toast daily can save a gain of 6 pounds.

And omit either just one scrambled egg or two slices of bacon once a week and you have a saving in either case of 1½ pounds over a year.

And consider other examples in Table 1.

ITEM	OMIT JUST	HOW OFTEN	WEIGHT GAIN SAVED PER YEAR
Bread stuffing	½ serving	once a week	1 lb.
Pork and beans	½ serving	once a week	2½ lbs.
Rice	½ serving	once a week	1 lb.
Creamed cottage cheese	1 cup	once a week	3 lbs.
Avocado	½	once a week	2½ lbs.
Yogurt, plain	1 cup	once a week	2 lbs.
Whole roasted peanuts	¼ cup	once a week	3 lbs.
Potato chips	10	once a week	1½ lbs.
Crackers	2	twice a week	1 lb.
Cheese	1 ounce	once a week	1½ lbs.
Ice cream soda	1	once a week	5 lbs.
Chocolate cake with frosting	1 slice	once a week	4 lbs.
Sugar	1 teaspoon	once a day	1½ lbs.
Doughnut	1	once a week	2 lbs.
Pie	½ slice	twice a week	3½ lbs.
Jam or jelly	1 tablespoon	twice a week	1½ lbs.

SIGNIFICANT SUBSTITUTIONS

Often, the caloric content of foods of similar type can vary greatly. And substituting the lower-calorie item for the higher-calorie can mean significant savings.

For example, use of a cup of consommé (25 calories) in place of a cup of split-pea soup (200 calories) saves 175 calories. And you can make an equal saving by substituting Manhattan clam chowder (1 cup = 100 calories) for New England clam chowder (1 cup = 275 calories).

Eat 1 cup of plain popcorn (about 65 calories) instead of the buttered kind (172 calories) and you save 107 calories.

A boiled egg (85 calories) replacing a fried egg (120 calories) saves 35 calories.

And if a cup of whole milk, with 3.5 percent fat and 165

calories, is replaced by a cup of skim milk, with 85 calories, the saving comes to 80 calories.

Table 2 shows the savings possible with other substitutions.

TABLE 2: SUBSTITUTION SAVINGS

For	Substitute	And save this many calories
SNACKS		
10 nuts, mixed (94 calories)	10 very thin pretzel sticks (10)	84
10 potato chips (108 calories)	10 cheese tidbits (20)	88
6 Ritz or Triscuit crackers (120 calories)	6 raw carrot sticks (18)	102
3 tablespoons roasted peanuts (258 calories)	3 tablespoons raisins (87)	171
MEAT, FISH, POULTRY		
½ fried chicken (464 calories)	6 oz. broiled chicken (257)	207
3 oz. hamburger and bun (400 calories)	3 oz. roast beef and roll (300)	100
3 strips bacon (144 calories)	1 slice Canadian bacon (65)	79
6 oz. fried shrimp (380 calories)	6 oz. boiled shrimp (200)	180
6 oz. breaded fried perch (384 calories)	6 oz. broiled fish (288)	96
BREADS, CEREALS		
1 slice bread (60 calories)	2 pieces Melba toast (40)	20
½ cup fried rice (175 calories)	½ cup plain rice (70)	105

54

For	Substitute	And save this many calories
BREADS, CEREALS		
½ cup granola-type cereal (500 calories)	1 cup corn flakes (95)	405
½ cup lasagne (175 calories)	½ cup plain noodles (95)	80
VEGETABLES		
½ cup potato salad (125 calories)	½ cup raw-vegetable salad without dressing (20)	105
20 French-fries (270 calories)	1 baked potato, medium (90)	180
½ cup corn kernels (70 calories)	½ cup cooked green beans (14)	56
DESSERTS, SWEET SNACKS		
2 chocolate-chip cookies (104 calories)	2 vanilla wafers (34)	70
1 piece chocolate cake with icing (400 calories)	1 piece angel cake (121)	279
½ cup bread pudding with raisins (210 calories)	½ cup plain gelatin dessert (81)	129
⅙ apple pie (410 calories)	1 sweetened baked apple (160)	250
½ cup Brown Betty (211 calories)	1 medium apple (88)	123
½ cup chocolate ice cream (150 calories)	½ cup orange ice (72)	78

7
Food and Preparation Guidelines

Obviously, there are foods that contain more calories than others, even very much more.

But that's not the whole story.

Some foods high in calories aren't always that way to begin with; preparation makes them so.

Some items are high in calories—yet don't satisfy hunger.

Some foods are quite low in calories—yet do appease.

Here are guidelines and insights which I can recommend because many of my patients—and their parents—have found them most helpful.

FOOD PREPARATION

How foods are prepared can be of major importance. Make it a point to avoid, or at least minimize, increasing the calories in foods through the addition of fats, coatings, or high-calorie sauces. These may be pleasing to the palate, but they are not necessary for satisfying hunger or stimulating the appetite.

All items added to food for flavor should have as few calories as possible. (See Condiments, below.)

Avoid frying in oil. Fry or scramble eggs in a nonstick pan that does not require the addition of fat. Recall from Chapter 6 that omitting just a single pat of butter or margarine daily can, all by itself, prevent the gain of 3½ pounds in the course of a year.

Breading is permissible on occasion—but then only when a serving of bread is removed from the rest of the day's menus to make up for it.

As a general rule, it can be remarkably helpful to do more broiling, boiling, and roasting rather than frying or sautéeing.

BEVERAGES

Not only soft drinks but juices and even milk can add many calories to the diet without satisfying hunger.

Allow either one glass of low-fat or skim milk or one glass of juice with each meal and for a bedtime snack. All other drinks during the day and at meals should be plain water, sparkling water, or unsweetened tea.

CONDIMENTS

Mustard, horseradish, vinegar, and spices such as pepper, paprika, basil, garlic, curry will not add significantly to the calories in a meal. Salt has no calories but should be used in moderation because of its possible role in elevating blood pressure.

Mayonnaise, salad dressing, ketchup, tomato sauce, and sugar will add calories and should be used on a limited basis. There are low-fat mayonnaise preparations on the market and they are preferable to regular mayonnaise, but they still add calories.

STARCHES

All starches should be eaten in measured quantities.

There is no need to eliminate potatoes or rice or bread from the diet, but a meal should have only one serving of starch:

bread—1 slice (unless the meal is a sandwich,
            in which case 2 slices);
or rice, peas, beans, corn or pasta—½ cup;
or potato—1 small;
or muffin or roll—1.

Do not add fat in the form of butter or margarine.

Vegetables

High-fiber green vegetables and other vegetables such as cauliflower and mushrooms can be eaten almost without limit. Green salads make an excellent filler at mealtime. Eaten raw, such vegetables also provide crispy, refreshing snacks. One snack that happens to be a favorite of mine is sliced fresh mushrooms lightly salted and then broiled.

The list that follows consists of vegetables that can be eaten virtually without limit. They should be steamed, boiled, or raw.

Asparagus	Chicory	Peppers, green or red
Broccoli	Cucumbers	Radishes
Brussels sprouts	Eggplant	Sauerkraut
Cabbage	Escarole	Squash, summer
Carrots	Lettuce	String beans
Cauliflower	Mushrooms	Watercress
Celery	Okra	Zucchini

Greens of: beet, chard, collard, dandelion, kale, mustard, spinach, turnip.

Tomatoes, beets, onions, and winter squash should be eaten less freely but are still relatively low in calories.

Starchy vegetables, listed above in the section on starches, should be limited to one portion at meals.

Meats

Meats should be boiled or broiled.

All visible fat should be trimmed off before cooking. And skin should be removed from poultry before eating.

Red meats such as beef and lamb should be limited to two meals a week. White meats, such as veal and chicken, are lower in calories and cholesterol. Portions should be limited to three to four ounces per meal.

Fish

Fish such as flounder, pike, and haddock are very low in calories when baked or broiled. Gefülte fish also is low in calories, but the jelly it is packed in is not.

Tuna is higher in calories, but is still a good bet if you get it packed in water rather than oil.

Shellfish—lobster, shrimp, and scallops—are also low in calories if prepared simply.

Take advantage of the low-calorie, high-nutrition benefits of fish and shellfish in several meals a week without having seconds.

DAIRY

Eggs are high in protein and low in calories—a good source of nutrition; but since egg yolk is high in cholesterol and eggs are used in many prepared foods, most experts recommend eggs at only 3 meals per week.

Milk products are high in nutrition—and fat. The low-fat version of milk products should be used, since the removal of the fat content halves the calories.

One of the great myths of dieting is that yogurt and cheese are diet foods. Even a single serving of low-fat fruit yogurt contains 240 to 260 calories. A 1-ounce slice of cheese contains 100 calories and is not usually enough for a meal. On the other hand, a half-cup scoop of low-fat cottage cheese has only 90 calories and is a satisfying portion.

FRUITS

Fruits are a source of carbohydrate. They are rich in fructose, a natural sugar.

Cantaloupe is an excellent fruit choice as part of a meal, since half a cantaloupe contains only 40 calories—and with the addition of a scoop of low-fat cottage cheese can make a refreshing and satisfying 130-calorie lunch.

Berries in measured quantities (½ cup) or a single fruit, fresh or dried, is an enjoyable snack, but not to be eaten without limit.

FATS

Added fats such as butter or margarine, even a low-fat version, should be kept to a bare minimum. The same is true for oil. Fatty foods include nuts, cream, cream cheese, dressings, and bacon.

The peanut butter–and–jelly sandwich (285 calories)—one of childhood's great delights—is primarily fat and carbohydrate, with some protein. A reasonable limit for those children who cannot live without it is one sandwich a week.

CANDIES, CAKE, AND COOKIES

These are not part of most diets because they are concentrated calories that satisfy only cravings, not hunger. A small chocolate bar, for example, may contain 155 calories; a medium-size cookie, 75; a plain doughnut, 135.

Candies, cake, and cookies should be reserved for special occasions and eaten in moderation. Special treats become more special when they are not part of the daily bill of fare.

8
Diet Exchange Lists:
Valuable Tools to Work With

Suppose you could find some relatively simple means that would allow you to achieve, at once, all the following:
• Plan menus that incorporate a specific number of calories;
• Beyond that, ensure that meals are balanced in terms of appropriate amounts of protein, carbohydrate, and fat;
• Ensure variety—and not only to maintain interest but also to provide known essential vitamins and minerals along with other nutrients that are fully as vital but still remain to be discovered.

Those, in fact, are the purposes of the diet exchange lists, along with the daily food plan which we will be going into in this chapter.

They can help you, as an older child, in designing your own diet—or as a parent, in designing a diet for a younger child: in both cases, an individualized diet to meet specific needs and preferences, likely to be far more effective and preferable than any handed-down stock diet.

They can help, too, by providing insights into foods and their makeup that, in common with most people, you may never have had before.

THE LISTS

As you see in the Table of Diet Exchange Lists on pages 62–68, there are six exchange lists, along with a seventh supplemental list which shows foods that can be eaten as desired.

The six lists are for milk exchanges, vegetable exchanges, fruit exchanges, bread exchanges, meat exchanges, and fat exchanges.

Foods in the lists are grouped according to their nutrient similarities, and in any one list all the foods shown are equal in value to each other in the amounts indicated.

Thus, for example, ½ cup of any vegetable shown in the vegetable exchanges list will contain 5 grams of carbohydrate and 2 grams of protein and will provide 25 calories.

And in the fruit exchanges list, either 1 small apple or half a small banana or ⅓ cup of pineapple juice, for example, will contain 10 grams of carbohydrate and provide 40 calories.

And in fact, the term "exchange" is appropriate because a serving of food within a list can be exchanged for a serving of another food within that list, depending upon individual preference, while ensuring the same nutrient values and calorie amounts.

Table of Diet Exchange Lists

List 1: Milk Exchanges

One exchange provides:
carbohydrate, 12 grams; protein, 8 grams; fat, trace; and 80 calories.

FOOD	QUANTITY FOR 1 EXCHANGE
Buttermilk, skim	1 cup
Nonfat dry milk, mixed according to directions	1 cup
Nonfat dry milk powder	¼ cup
Skim milk	1 cup
Yogurt, plain, skim-milk	1 cup
1%-fat milk (provided you omit ½ fat exchange)	1 cup
2%-fat milk (provided you omit 1 fat exchange)	1 cup

62

FOOD	QUANTITY FOR 1 EXCHANGE
Whole milk (provided you omit 2 fat exchanges)	1 cup
Yogurt, plain, whole-milk (provided you omit 2 fat exchanges)	1 cup

LIST 2: VEGETABLE EXCHANGES

One exchange provides:
carbohydrate, 5 grams; protein, 2 grams; and 25 calories.
One exchange = ½ cup.

Asparagus
Bean sprouts
Beets
Broccoli
Brussels sprouts
Cabbage
Carrots
Cauliflower
Celery
Cucumbers
Eggplant
Green pepper

Greens:
Beet
Chard
Collard
Dandelion
Kale
Mustard
Spinach
Turnip
Mushrooms
Okra
Onions

Rhubarb
Rutabaga
Sauerkraut
String beans,
    green or yellow
Summer squash
Tomatoes
Tomato juice
Turnips
Vegetable-juice
    cocktail
Zucchini

NOTE: *Starchy vegetables are in the Bread Exchanges list.*

LIST 3: FRUIT EXCHANGES

One exchange provides:
carbohydrate, 10 grams; and 40 calories.

FOOD	QUANTITY FOR 1 EXCHANGE
Apple	1 small
Apple juice	⅓ cup
Applesauce	½ cup
Apricots, fresh	2 medium
Apricots, dried	4 halves

FOOD	QUANTITY FOR 1 EXCHANGE
Banana	½ small
Berries (boysenberries, blackberries, raspberries, strawberries)	1 cup
Blueberries	⅔ cup
Cantaloupe	¼ (6")
Cherries	10 large
Dates	2
Figs, fresh	2 large
Figs, dried	1 small
Fruit cocktail	½ cup
Grapefruit	½ small
Grapefruit juice	½ cup
Grapes	12
Grape juice	¼ cup
Honeydew melon	⅛ (7")
Mandarin oranges	¾ cup
Mango	½ small
Nectarine	1 small
Orange	1 small
Orange juice	½ cup
Papaya	⅓ medium
Peach	1 medium
Pear	1 small
Pineapple	½ cup
Pineapple juice	⅓ cup
Plums	2 medium
Prunes, dried	2
Prune juice	¼ cup
Raisins	2 tablespoons
Tangerine	1 large
Watermelon	1 cup

NOTE: *Fruits are eaten fresh, dried, frozen, or canned without sugar or syrup.*

LIST 4: BREAD EXCHANGES
(includes bread, cereal, starchy vegetables)
One exchange provides:
carbohydrate, 15 grams; protein, 2 grams; and 68
calories.

FOOD	QUANTITY FOR 1 EXCHANGE
Bread	1 slice
Bagel	½
Biscuit, roll	1 (2″)
Bun (hamburger)	½
Corn bread	1½″ cube
English muffin	½
Muffin	1 (2″)
Cake, angel or sponge, without icing	1½″ cube (1/20 of 10″ cake)
Cereal, cooked	½ cup
Cereal, dry (flakes or puffed)	¾ cup
Cornstarch	2 tablespoons
Crackers, graham	2 (2½″ square)
Crackers, oyster	20 (½ cup)
Crackers, round	6
Crackers, saltine	5
Crackers, variety	5 small
Flour	2½ tablespoons
Matzo	1 (6″)
Popcorn, popped, unbuttered	1 cup
Rice or grits, cooked	½ cup
Spaghetti, macaroni, or noodles, cooked	½ cup
Starchy vegetables:	
Beans, baked, without pork	¼ cup
Beans (lima, navy, etc.), dry, cooked	½ cup
Corn	⅓ cup
Corn on the cob	½ medium ear
Parsnips	⅔ cup
Peas (split, etc.), dry, cooked	½ cup
Potatoes, sweet or yams, fresh	¼ cup
Potatoes, white, baked or boiled	1 (2″)
Potatoes, white, mashed	½ cup

LIST 5: MEAT EXCHANGES
(includes cheese, fish, and other proteins)

One exchange provides:
protein, 7 grams; fat, 3 grams; and 55 calories.

FOOD	QUANTITY FOR 1 EXCHANGE
Lean meats and poultry, no skin	1 ounce (4" × 2" × ¼")
Fish, any fresh or frozen	1 ounce
Fish and shellfish:	
canned salmon, tuna, mackerel, crab, lobster	¼ cup
clams, oysters, scallops, shrimp	5 or 1 ounce
sardines, drained	3
Cheese, less than 5% butterfat	1 ounce
Cheese, cottage, low-fat	¼ cup

NOTE: *For the following foods—and also for medium-fat meats—count an additional ½ fat exchange per portion to be omitted from the daily food plan.*

Cottage cheese, creamed	¼ cup
Cheese:	
mozzarella, ricotta, farmer's, Neufchâtel	1 ounce
Parmesan	3 tablespoons
Egg	1

NOTE: *For the following foods—and also for high-fat meats, duck, spareribs—count an additional 1 fat exchange per portion to be omitted from the daily food plan.*

Cheese, cheddar	1 ounce
Cold cuts, 4½" × ⅛"	1 slice
Frankfurter	1 small
Peanut butter *(count 2 additional fat exchanges per portion to be omitted from the daily food plan)*	2 tablespoons

List 6: Fat Exchanges

One exchange provides:
fat, 5 grams; and 45 calories.

FOOD	QUANTITY FOR 1 EXCHANGE
Avocado	⅛ (4")
Bacon, crisp	1 slice
Butter or margarine	1 teaspoon
Cream:	
Half and half	3 tablespoons
Heavy, 40%	1 tablespoon
Light, 20%	2 tablespoons
Sour	2 tablespoons
Cream cheese	1 tablespoon
Dressing:	
French	1 tablespoon
Mayonnaise	1 teaspoon
Roquefort	2 teaspoons
Nuts	6 small
Oil or cooking fat	1 teaspoon
Olives	5 small

SPECIAL NOTE:

Any time an instruction for a food in any of the preceding six lists calls for counting one or more additional fat exchanges, that number of fat exchanges must be omitted from the daily food plan for each such portion of food chosen.

You can, if you like, consume all of an allotted exchange as one food. For example, when the Daily Food Plan (see below) allows 6 bread exchanges, you can choose 6 slices of bread—or you can fill the allotment with different foods such as 1 cup of cooked cereal, 1 cup of noodles, and 2 slices of bread, which add up to 6 bread exchanges.

You can also distribute exchanges for any given meal according to your preferences—but allotted meat, fat, and bread exchanges should usually be used at each meal.

Seasonings: Salt, cinnamon, garlic, lemon, mustard, mint, nutmeg, parsley, pepper, vanilla, vinegar, etc.

Other items: coffee or tea (without sugar or cream), fat-free broth or bouillon, unflavored gelatin, sour or dill pickles, cranberries, chicory, Chinese cabbage, endive, escarole, lettuce, parsley, radishes, watercress. *The vegetables are eaten raw.*

THE DAILY FOOD PLAN

By using the exchange lists in conjunction with a daily food plan, you can plan menus to provide a desired number of calories per day.

And most importantly, this type of meal planning differs from just counting calories in that it also takes into account the composition of foods and balances the diet, allowing for healthy variety as well.

Here is a daily food plan chart which shows the number of exchanges per day for foods in each of the six exchange lists depending upon desired number of calories, ranging from 1,100 to 2,700, per day.

DAILY FOOD PLAN

	Number of exchanges per day							
CALORIES	1,100	1,300	1,400	1,600	2,000	2,200	2,500	2,700
FOOD EXCHANGE LIST								
Milk	2	2	2	3	3	3	3	3
Fruit	2	3	3	3	4	4	4	5
Vegetable	1	1	2	3	3	3	3	3
Bread	6	7	7	8	11	12	15	16
Meat	2	2	3	3	3	4	5	6
Fat	7	9	9	10	14	15	16	17

If the daily food plan is followed, using the portions allowed in the exchange list, the diet will be very desirably balanced, consisting of approximately 50 percent carbohydrate, 30 percent fat, and 20 percent protein.

USING A PLAN

As an example of how to use a daily food plan, let's go back to the 9-year-old boy we mentioned in Chapter 2 whose weight could be brought into line by reduction of his food intake to between 2,200 and 2,700 calories.

Let's say we choose the lower figure—2,200 calories. A glance at the daily food plan chart under the 2,200-calories heading shows the number of exchanges for the six food lists.

The boy can, as we see, have 3 milk exchanges. Generally, the three should be distributed through three meals, one at each meal. But there is room for flexibility.

Perhaps there is one meal where no item from the milk exchange list may be wanted. For example, you may be having meat for dinner and you would prefer fruit juice as a beverage rather than milk. You can then plan to use two milk exchanges for breakfast and one for lunch, or vice versa, or you may prefer to have a milk exchange as a snack.

You are allowed 4 fruit exchanges for a day. You can divide those up any way you like—perhaps two for breakfast and one each at the other two meals. Or you may use some of the fruit exchanges for snacking. Fruits make good snacks, but they do have to be taken into account because of their caloric content —unlike the high-fiber, low-calorie vegetables such as chicory, escarole, radishes, and watercress in List 7.

You have the same flexibility with exchanges from the other lists when it comes to setting up your menu for a day.

9
Design Your Own Diet

You may be wondering why I did not write an exact diet plan accompanied by sets of menus—all very neat, standardized, well ordered.

There are three reasons why not.

For one thing, I am convinced that if I can provide you with pertinent, succinct information about nutrition as it applies to effective weight control, then no matter where you may be and what food may be available, you will be able to make the right decision about what to eat without having to worry about following some exact diet plan. Your understanding and good eating habits should become a natural part of your decision process.

Secondly, children of different ages, different sizes, different growth rates, different caloric requirements, and coming from different family backgrounds certainly cannot all benefit from some one standard regimen. To meet the needs of all kinds of growing, changing children, there must be great flexibility.

And thirdly, I wanted this book to be useful for children who don't want to eat, like automatons, say, grapefruit for breakfast every Tuesday.

Now that you have read the preceding chapters of this book, you have all the information necessary to design a diet that will meet your specific needs and food preferences. The only kinds of diets not provided for in this book are fad diets and highly restrictive diets that promise quick weight loss.

I strongly oppose and discourage the use of any rapid-weight-loss diets for growing children; I do not think they are sound for growth, and they do not teach good eating habits that one can depend upon for the rest of life.

A FIRST STEP

Now, to design your personalized diet, the first thing to do is examine your eating habits. You can do this best if you kept a log as recommended in Chapter 6.

Take a look at the foods you eat and see which exchange lists they are in.

Do you eat many foods from the fat exchange list—or many fatty meats?

Are many ingredients from the fat exchange list used in the preparation of the foods you eat?

Do you, primarily, eat starchy vegetables, those found in the bread exchange list, or do you eat mostly the high-fiber, low-calorie vegetables?

Do you depend upon protein and starchy foods to fill you up at mealtime, or do you eat fresh salads and lots of low-calorie vegetables as part of your meal to help fill you up?

Once you have answered these questions, you know some of the eating habits you need to change.

THE "UNDOING" FOODS

Look again at your log.

Is there a particular food that is your undoing at mealtime or when you have a snack? If there is and it is not a nutritious food, remove it from your diet and never eat it except when you allow yourself a special treat.

A typical example would be something like potato chips. Why potato chips? Potatoes are nutritious; they contain many nutrients. But for potato chips, potatoes are peeled, sliced thin, fried in oil, and salted. So to get some of the nutritional benefits of a potato, you are consuming something that has a lot of salt and fat in it. And generally, one potato is enough for most of us—but when we sit down with a bag of potato chips, we are pretty certain to consume more than the equivalent of a single potato before we are satisfied. Salty foods tend to make you crave more of them.

So I would pick potato chips as a food that starts out from a good nutritional base but then has been turned into something not soundly nutritious. This is not to say that you should never have a potato chip—but potato chips are not, to my mind, an ideal food.

Nuts, on the other hand, can be considered somewhat nutritious since they contain protein. But they are a high-fat food, and again, if you salt them, you turn them into a junk food which you sit and eat in large quantities, adding much fat and needless salt to your diet.

Another example of a nonnutritious food is the candy bar. I am far more concerned about candy bars than I am about other childhood snacks such as cookies.

Candy bars contain a lot of fat. They are not primarily carbohydrate. And in fact, physicians often have to educate diabetics that a candy bar is not what they are to take when they become hypoglycemic. In addition, candy bars, along with their fat content, contain sweeteners, and I think that anything excessively sweet tends to increase the desire to eat more of it. And so I put candy bars in the category of junk foods.

I am less adamant about food items like cookies when eaten in moderation. A cookie can be somewhat like a breadstuff if it is not excessively sweet. An oatmeal cookie can contain whole grain and can have fruit in it, and can be a nutritious food.

But we must realize that once we sweeten something, we are going to increase the desire to eat it—often to excess.

TREATS

If you tend to have cravings for a particular nutritious food, decide right now how much of it would be reasonable to eat for a meal or snack. Set a daily or weekly limit—and stick to that limit.

Suppose there is a food you feel you must eat which is not discussed in Chapter 7 or is not in the exchange lists in Chapter 8. In all likelihood, it is a food high in calories. If you wish to eat it on a regular basis, check for it in Appendix D, or use a calorie counter to determine the food's content of carbohydrate, protein, and fat as well as calories. Then go to the exchange lists and figure out which foods from your regular daily diet would be equivalent and eliminate them the day you eat your special food.

For example, suppose you want pizza. It is not a recommended food in most diets. An average slice of pizza provides 240 calories and contains 14 grams of protein, 9 grams of fat, and 25 grams of carbohydrate. That slice would be approximately the equivalent of 2 ounces of lean meat (containing 14 grams of protein and 6 grams of fat), *plus* one slice of bread (with 15 grams of carbohydrate and 2 grams of protein), *plus* 1 fruit (with 10 grams of carbohydrate), *plus* ½ teaspoonful of mayonnaise or margarine (with 2½ grams of fat).

In short, multiple foods would have to be omitted from your regular meals to compensate for that slice of pizza.

The point is that you can eat any kind of food—but you must plan for it. Often, you have to give up too many things just to eat one special food, so it is usually best to reserve that food for a special treat.

Most of us like to have a special treat on weekends or when we go out or to a party. The once-weekly treat is not likely to destroy your diet; but you must be sensible.

If you have a special dinner, don't follow it with a fattening dessert. If it's dessert you crave when you're out, try to keep your meal within the guidelines of your diet. If you really expect to go far outside your diet guidelines for a given meal, see if you can borrow from the other meals of the day; but do not skip meals or go hungry, because you're likely to eat even more if you're starved.

YOUR DIET—WITH AND WITHOUT EXACT GUIDELINES

You know what your objective is—and it is not to lose a lot of weight quickly, at possibly high cost in health and normal growth and without establishing a healthy pattern of eating. Rather, you want to maintain your weight; keep it under control where it is; add no more pounds, so that at some point, as you grow, it becomes a normal, slim, healthy weight for you.

You may or may not be able to achieve your goal without exact food guidelines and attention to calories.

Individual circumstances, of course, vary. It is sometimes possible to stop further weight gain by making use of only the "tricks" of dieting described in Chapter 6. Go over that chapter again.

Perhaps just learning to eat more slowly than you now do, using the techniques indicated in Chapter 6, giving satiety a chance to set in earlier at each meal, can be enough for you.

Perhaps the "omission maneuvers" noted in Chapter 6 will work well. For some, they add up to significant savings in pounds gained. And that is also true for the "significant substitutions" described in the same chapter.

Perhaps several of these techniques combined can suffice for you.

If not, you can develop daily or weekly menus for the number of calories you need, using the daily food plan and the exchange lists in Chapter 8. And note: to design a lower-fat, higher-protein diet, you can replace 5 fat exchanges with 4 meat exchanges on the daily food plan (or a proportionate amount, such as 2½ fat to 2 meat or 10 fat to 8 meat) and then go to the exchange lists to make your menus. Here is the lower-fat food plan arrived at by this method.

LOWER-FAT DAILY FOOD PLAN

Number of exchanges per day

CALORIES	1,100	1,300	1,400	1,600	2,000	2,200	2,500	2,700
FOOD EXCHANGE LIST								
Milk	2	2	2	3	3	3	3	3
Fruit	2	3	3	3	4	4	4	5
Vegetable	1	1	2	3	3	3	3	3
Bread	6	7	7	8	11	12	15	16
Meat	6	6	7	7	7	8	9	10
Fat	2	4	4	5	9	10	11	12

START NOW

You're ready now to begin to bring your weight under control.

Weigh yourself—and record the weight.

And after that, weigh yourself once or twice a week. Many people drop a few pounds at first because of loss of excess water. If you don't lose, don't be discouraged. Remember, your goal is zero weight gain.

Some fluctuation of your weight is bound to occur from time to time. If your weight should ever reach 4 pounds more than your starting weight, then your diet needs to be revised in favor of lower caloric intake.

No need to feel sorry for yourself. On the contrary, you have every reason to congratulate yourself.

You're not embarking on any regimen of torture and deprivation. You're not following in the footsteps of many adults who should know better but never seem to learn, who go on one fad diet after another, depriving and torturing themselves for days or weeks at a time, quickly losing some weight—only to regain it promptly; then repeating the deprivation and torture with still another fad diet, and going through this over and over again.

You will be eating well, nutritiously, healthily. And if you eat a little less overall, and in particular of some foods, you'll nonetheless come to enjoy what you eat and probably enjoy it even more than before.

Try it and you will see.

10
Exercise

It's not just a mere add-on, something that may be mildly helpful. On the contrary, there may be nothing more important—more to-the-point—that you can do for an overweight child than to encourage physical activity.

And that includes participation in games and sports he or she may never have tried before or may have tried and given up on.

Despite any myths to the contrary, regular physical activity can make a tremendous difference for weight control. Lack of activity is not just *a* factor in excessive weight gain; it is a significant influence.

Moreover, activity—exercise—has other major values.

We've seen adult Americans become increasingly aware recently of those values—for physical, mental, and emotional health as well as for weight control. They apply no less to children—and they can be lifelong values.

For your encouragement to be effective, thoughtful effort —more than mere urging—may be needed. And we'll consider that. But before doing so, let's look at *all* that exercise has to offer any child, and especially an overweight one.

PHYSICAL HEALTH

It's an old saying—with new meaning today. The child is, indeed, "father of the man (or woman)"—and in terms of

76

physical well-being as well as healthy personality.

Physical health problems, once considered strictly adult problems, are now turning out to have their beginnings in childhood.

For example, high blood pressure and elevated blood-fat levels—two of the major risk factors for heart and blood-vessel disease—are common among adult Americans, with hypertension alone affecting at least one-third of American men and women.

But are they strictly adult problems?

On the contrary, with recent intensification of studies on children, both conditions have begun to be found at early ages.

By high school age, according to studies by Professor Thomas B. Gilliam of the University of Michigan, close to half of youngsters show evidence of one or more risk factors.

And now engaged in a long-term study to determine to what extent physical activity can help, Gilliam is finding marked reductions in blood fats occurring within 3 months after institution of an activity program.

Other research indicates that vigorous physical activity can help to some extent in controlling blood pressure.

Still other studies have found, as you might expect, that exercise can increase general muscular strength and endurance and, beyond that, may in time help to overcome easy fatigue or feelings of listlessness. Exercise also has proved valuable in correcting postural defects.

MENTAL ACHIEVEMENT

In the Research Digest it publishes, the President's Council on Physical Fitness and Sports has considered the evidence from many studies of the relationship between fitness and mental achievement.

"More studies," the Council reports, "produced positive relationships between physical-motor traits and mental achievement than resulted in nil or negative results. It may be contended that a person's general learning potential for a given level of intelligence is increased or decreased in accordance with his or her degree of physical fitness."

To state this in less formal terms, it appears that whatever the intelligence level of an individual, his or her ability to learn may be favorably influenced by physical fitness.

EMOTIONAL HEALTH

Children, like adults, face stressful situations. Unless they develop means of properly coping with stress, they, like adults, can become tense, anxious, depressed—and also like adults, they can develop stress-induced headaches, intestinal disturbances, skin rashes, and other disorders.

As more and more intelligent adults are learning, physical activity is perhaps the best means of dealing with otherwise disturbing stress reactions—more relaxing and certainly more healthful than a tranquilizer.

You have probably found, in your own experience, that if you're bothered by a problem, wound up, perhaps temporarily frustrated, you may experience a violent need to get up and move about, *not* to sit still. And you may have discovered, too, that it's difficult if not impossible to stay all wound up if you play a game of tennis or jog or take a brisk walk or perhaps play ball with the kids.

That physical activity seems relaxing is everyday experience. And a possible reason for this, based on the concept of stress, has been suggested: When, in response to a stressful situation, you become tense and anxious, the adrenal glands atop the kidneys produce hormone secretions designed to prepare you to fight or flee. In effect, you're mobilized for physical action.

What goes on is a carryover from the time of our ancient ancestors who became tense and anxious in situations of physical emergency—confronted, for example, with a fierce animal or dangerous storm or other natural peril. To live, they had to react quickly, either by standing up to the peril or by running from it. The increased adrenal-gland outpourings of hormones gave them the extra energy for this.

Today, we are rarely confronted with such emergencies. Much more often, when we become tense and anxious, it's because of a problem or pressure we can't respond to by fighting or fleeing. Instead, we're likely to sit and become tense and wound up.

78

We're wound up with unused energy that churns around inside, making us uncomfortable as we sit, unable to direct the energy outward as our ancestors did in very different types of stress-provoking situations.

But we can work off the energy—and much of the tension —by physical activity.

No wonder that the recently released U.S. Surgeon General's Report called "Healthy People" and subtitled "Health Promotion and Disease Prevention" could view exercise enthusiastically.

"People who exercise regularly," the Report observed, "report that they feel better, have more energy, often require less sleep. Regular exercisers often lose weight as well as improve muscular strength and flexibility. Many also experience psychological benefits including enhanced self-esteem, greater self-reliance, decreased anxiety, and relief from mild depression."

EXERCISE AND WEIGHT CONTROL

One widely held misconception is that exercise has little to contribute to weight control because it would take huge amounts of time and effort to burn up enough calories to have any significant effect on weight.

But that can hardly be true—and it definitely is not.

Consider that the very active—among them, ditchdiggers and other laborers, athletes, and soldiers in the field—may take in as many as 5,000 to 6,000 calories a day, twice as much as average or even more, and yet gain no weight.

In one classical trial, investigators had a group of college students deliberately double their usual food intake, going from 3,000 to 6,000 calories a day, while at the same time greatly increasing their exercise and other physical activity. No weight gain.

Putting on a pound of excess weight requires taking in 3,500 calories more than expended. Losing a pound requires the reverse: an expenditure of 3,500 calories more than taken in. But it isn't a matter of doing it in a day or a week.

If exercise is increased enough to burn up an extra 200 calories a day, that would mean 73,000 calories in a year—

enough to lose 20 excess pounds or prevent that much of a gain. And burning up those extra calories could involve, for example, no more than 20 minutes of handball, swimming (at 40 yards a minute), fast cycling, or jogging.

Moreover, evidence from some recent studies suggests that exercise effects may continue beyond the exercise period. During vigorous physical activity, body processes increase their pace—and it appears that there is a gradual, not sudden, slowing of the pace afterward. Which means that energy (calorie) use continues at a stepped-up pace for a time after exercise stops.

Worth noting too: numerous studies have looked at differences between the obese and people of normal weight in terms of food intake and activity patterns—and many of the obese have been found to eat no more than people of normal weight but to be much less physically active.

Some years ago, when Dr. Jean Mayer and a team of Harvard investigators compared the caloric intake and physical activity of obese and normal schoolgirls, they found that most of the overweight girls weren't consuming more food than the normal girls but they were spending two-thirds less time in physical activity.

As part of the Harvard study, a series of 29,000 short (3-second) movies, taken every 3 minutes, of obese and normal girls as they engaged in various physical activities were analyzed. The time spent in motion by the obese girls and the caloric cost of the motion proved to be much less than the corresponding values for the nonobese.

For example, when they were playing tennis, normal girls were in motion more than 85 percent of the time; on the other hand, the obese girls were standing still 60 percent of the time. In volleyball, girls of normal weight were in motion, on average, half the time; the obese girls were standing still 85 percent of the time.

There is also another common misconception: that you can't win with exercise; it's self-defeating since it increases appetite and thus is likely to increase rather than hold down weight.

Yet many scientific studies have disproved that notion.

Report both the Committee on Exercise and Physical Fitness of the American Medical Association and the President's Council on Physical Fitness: "It is true that a lean person in good condition may eat more following increased activity, but his exercise will burn up the extra calories he consumes. But the obese person does not react the same way. Only when an obese person exercises to excess will appetite increase. Because he has large stores of fat, moderate exercise does not stimulate appetite. The difference between the response to exercise of fat and lean people is important."

AVERAGE ENERGY EXPENDITURES FOR VARIOUS PHYSICAL ACTIVITIES

LIGHT EXERCISE 4 calories/ minute	MODERATE EXERCISE 7 calories/ minute	HEAVY EXERCISE 10 calories/ minute
Dancing (slow step)	Badminton, singles	Calisthenics, vigorous
Golf	Cycling, 9½ miles per hour	Cycling, 12 miles per hour
Table Tennis	Dancing, fast step	Handball
Volleyball	Stationary cycling, moderate pace	Paddleball
Walking, 3 miles per hour	Swimming, 30 yards per minute	Squash
	Tennis, singles	Jogging
	Walking, 3½ miles per hour	Skipping rope
		Stationary cycling, fast pace
		Jogging in place
		Swimming, 40 yards per minute

ENCOURAGING ACTIVITY

Children, even at the youngest ages, have an inherent urge to be active.

81

Watch even a 6-month-old roll over one day; a few weeks later pull up to a standing position; soon start crawling; and a few weeks later even get up on hands and knees. Roll a ball toward the child and he or she returns it.

If you provide a young child with things to climb on and things to play with that require that the child move, there will be plenty of activity.

For an older child—one who already has well-developed balance and knows how to run and play—even calisthenics can be fun. But that will be true only if it is not something imposed.

In a family where mother or father or both get down on the floor at some given period during the day and exercise, kids will want to join in. And even if they can't do the situps and pushups parents may do to keep trim and in shape, they will want to try and will think it is fun, part of what the family does.

Children vary in the age at which they develop abilities to carry out certain activities, but as soon as the abilities are there, the activities can, and usually should, be encouraged.

Most youngsters can begin to ride a tricycle by age 3—and most can handle a bicycle, with or without training wheels, by age 6. Many children can learn to skate early on, although somebody may have to be available with a helping hand. By age 7 or 8, most kids can skate without holding on.

INTO SPORTS

Getting a youngster involved in a sport—if he has any interest in the sport—is probably the best way to guarantee some regularity of exercise.

But if your child is obese and has become sedentary at least in part because of the obesity and the accompanying reluctance to go out for any sport because of a fear of being shown up, he or she is hardly alone.

The problem is common but not insoluble.

The first thing that you, as a concerned parent, may need to do to encourage sports participation is find out a child's interests.

Most kids, just because they are kids, have at least an interest in some sports, even if the interest is limited to watching. If a youngster likes to watch some particular sport, he or she almost certainly has enough of an interest in it to warrant trying to get him or her involved in playing it.

The next step is to find out whether there is an organized program for that sport in which your child may fit. That can be no easy matter. An all-too-common problem with competitive sports is that obese youngsters—and many others who, for one reason or another, are less than top-notch—are left out.

Each year, 20 million American kids aged from 6 up play, or try to play, on organized sports teams. Two million want to play Little League baseball; 1 million, organized football; others are eager to play hockey or soccer, or to participate in swimming, track, or other activities.

Some benefit. But many are hurt. They are humiliated, their pride damaged. They make no teams. They are quickly eliminated. And the fat ones, of course, are among them— victims of overemphasis on a "winning is all" philosophy.

Perhaps no one has put it better than Dr. Thomas Tutko, a sports psychologist, cofounder of the Institute of Athletic Motivation at San Jose State University, and long a psychological consultant to many pro athletic teams, including the Los Angeles Rams, Pittsburgh Steelers, Dallas Cowboys, and Miami Dolphins.

In his book titled *Winning Is Everything—and Other American Myths*, coauthored with William Bruns, Tutko has written:

> We organize children's leagues, give them uniforms, hand out trophies, set up play-offs and all-star teams, send them to "bowl" games, and encourage them to compete at earlier and earlier ages.
>
> Many people would argue that this should be the purpose of sports—to strive for records, championships, Olympic teams, and professional careers. But how many million youngsters are we sacrificing along the way so that ten players can entertain us in a pro basketball game? How many people are we eliminating who love sports, but who never make the team because they're not going to be "winners"—they're too short, or too slow, or too weak.

And Dr. Tutko might well have included the "too fat."
He goes on to add:

The idea should be to encourage physical activity by every child, not to weed out those who are uncoordinated or untalented. Let's compete, play to win, but keep it all in perspective. Young athletes should see the thrill of competing, not simply winning; they should be judged by their effort, not just the end results or lack of results.

Certainly, an important part of getting your youngster participating in a sport in which he is interested is to assure him from the beginning that you are not looking for him to win.

And then you have to do some checking around and, hopefully, find a team coach whose philosophy is not to win, win, win, to the exclusion of all else.

That may be at least a little less difficult than it has been—thanks to growing concern among parents, physicians, educators, coaches, and others about the winning-is-all philosophy.

One indication of the potential turnabout is the Youth Basketball Association first set up in 1975 by many YMCAs. A league for both boys and girls, 8 to 18, with teams that always play against other teams in the same age or grade category, it was organized for the purpose of setting a new tone for youth programs throughout the United States and Canada.

And the program's philosophy is clear:
• YBA is for everybody, not just those who excel.
• It's fun. That's what games for kids should be all about.
• All players are involved equally in the game, regardless of ability.
• Winning is put in proper perspective.
• Emphasis is on development of basic skills in the sport, with players urged to develop these skills as far as their individual interests and abilities permit.
• The whole family can get involved as volunteers.

After YBA's first year of operation, *The Wall Street Journal* published this story about it:

Needham, Mass. —Bruce Skinner, age 10, likes his new basketball coach at the local YMCA. "The old coach only cared about winning," Bruce says. "Andy, the new coach, just wants us to have fun."

What Bruce doesn't know is that his former coach was fired for doing precisely the things Bruce disliked. He "over-emphasized competition and set a bad example," says Steve Fulford, 25, the Y physical education director who ordered the switch.

Few coaches expect to be replaced for trying too hard to win. Steve's decision, however, jibed perfectly with the unorthodox goals of Bruce's league and 350 other leagues in the Youth Basketball Association. Run by YMCAs nationwide, the YBA encourages boys and girls to concentrate on basketball skills and teamwork, not on winning. The Association's coaches, all volunteers, are trained to stress personal values. Players keep scorecards that measure sportsmanship, as well as skills like shooting and dribbling. One question asks, "How much of a team player am I?" and responses range from "ball hog" to "playmaker."

YBA coaches sometimes even bend the rules to prevent lopsided victories that would discourage losers. When the halftime score was 30 to 2 in a game at Milwaukee, the coaches decreed that the leading team had to complete five passes before each shot. The second-half scoring was even, so the losing team obviously benefitted from the five-pass rule. The league director said the winners also benefitted because they got to practice their passing. The Association goes out of its way to involve parents in the program. They meet at workshops with coaches and players four times each season to see films, hear speeches and discuss YBA goals.

Parents even receive a bit of sports advice for themselves. The YBA manual includes a personal scorecard for parents that discourages them from putting too much pressure on their children. The manual cautions that "being a 'support' without being a 'push' is one of the big challenges for parents."

Some coaches and parents fear that downgrading competition hurts the quality of play, but Mr. Stepanek thinks the opposite is true. "Over all, the quality of play improves," he says, "because kids with less ability and more sensitive egos do much better without the high pressure. Only the best players are helped by intense competition."

It was the National Basketball Players Association, the

union for players in the National Basketball Association, that first suggested YMCA leagues.

It may well be a significant indication of the growing realization of the real value of sports for kids that the suggestion for establishing YBA and continued support for it has come from NBA players.

"We all support this program and its goals," says John Havlicek, one of the NBA players. "We think it's important for *all* kids to have an opportunity to learn to play basketball, regardless of ability, size, or any other of the physical characteristics which often eliminate kids from playing the game."

OTHER ALTERNATIVES

If no YBA or its equivalent is available for your youngsters, and if your search for a team coach with the YBA type of philosophy proves fruitless, there are other possibilities.

One, of course, is to go out and try to organize neighborhood teams. That can be sticky if your own child has not been willing to go out and seek friends to play with, but it can be worth doing.

There are also activities your youngster can get into without need for other kids. Swimming is one of the best; it uses virtually all muscles. Nor does a child have to be on a team to ice-skate or roller-skate.

For that matter, if your youngster can be interested in tennis, it takes only one other person to play—and that person could very well be you if you're willing to take the time.

Almost any two-person sport can be played by parent and child until the child becomes good enough at it to begin to seek competitors of his or her own age. For a parent who wants to get more involved with a child's life in order to help, I would heartily recommend two-person sports as the place to begin.

Another fact is very much worth considering here: Some sports tend to have lifetime value; others do not.

Few adults play baseball, football, or basketball, for example. On the other hand, a U.S. Public Health Survey has found that America's top participant sport for adult men and women is swimming. And, obviously enough, there has been a great increase of interest in jogging, running, biking, and tennis.

You may well wish to introduce your child to those sports or others which can be enjoyed for a lifetime. They include handball, racquetball, paddleball, soccer, volleyball, cross-country skiing, skating, and squash.

And you might like to consider, too, that when the President's Council on Physical Fitness and Sports asked a group of experts to rate various forms of activity for health values—from the standpoint of heart and lung endurance, muscular strength and endurance, flexibility, balance, and general well-being (including weight control, sleep, digestion)—these were the ratings in descending order of value, from most helpful to least:

Jogging	Downhill skiing
Bicycling	Tennis
Swimming	Calisthenics
Skating	Walking
Handball/squash	Golf (with cart)
Cross-country skiing	Softball
Basketball	Bowling

11
Family Encouragement and Support

I learned it long ago in dealing with the overweight children brought to me in my office—and I pass it on because I am sure it can stand you and your overweight child in good stead.

Some adolescents are self-motivated to control their weight, and that's especially so among young ladies. But certainly not even all adolescents are.

And it's very rare that a younger child has the motivation.

Take a 6-, 7-, or 8-year-old who is fat. He may very well not care that he is fat. The only way in which his overweight comes to his attention at all may be that other people make him feel out of place. Because his size seems perfectly natural to him. He doesn't know how he got that way. He doesn't internalize the idea of wanting to look attractive. If his peers and others are bothering him, it's not his fault; everyone else is mean.

And the immediate response you may well get from a child when you tell him he must lose weight is "Aw! You mean I can't have snacks? I can't have cookies?" And if you tell him then, "No, you can't," that's it; you've lost him. He is not going to cooperate.

On the other hand, it can be an entirely different story if you start out with the premise that you mustn't attack the child head on, you mustn't emphasize his excessive weight— but rather, you must minimize it and then minimize the treatment.

You say to the child: "You are a little bit overweight. A little bit." And you show him the growth chart. He can't understand the chart.

But rather than looking at the child and pointing to his body and saying how fat a body he has, you have him look with you at the chart, and you say: "Well, you see here how we've plotted your height and weight, and how you compare with other children of your age, and you are a little overweight. And I think if you could be more the same weight as other children of your age and size, you would probably be happier. And if it weren't too hard to do, you would be glad to do it.

"Now, the trick is," you go on to say, "you don't have to lose any weight. You just have to be careful not to gain weight as quickly as you've been doing."

You go further: "You see, last year you weighed seven pounds less than you do now. And if you had not gained any weight instead of gaining seven pounds, you would be right about where you belong. Now, do you think it would be too difficult for you not to keep gaining as much weight?"

And most children can handle that idea. Most are likely to say, "Yes, I think I can do it."

You've won points because the child is willing to listen to what you have to say next.

The minute you attack, however, telling him something is wrong with him and you're going to change it, you've lost him. Because little kids are fragile when it comes to their self-image. They view things as being done to and for them because they don't see themselves as being very independent. And if you tell a child you're going to put him on a diet because he is fat, you're telling him, essentially, that he is bad and you are going to punish him.

Because—why *is* he fat? He overindulges. The basic American societal attitude toward fat people is "You are fat; you overindulge. If you must diet, you deserve to; it's your punishment."

You will not get a child's cooperation if that is how he interprets what you are saying.

So you defuse the situation. You deemphasize the idea that the child is fat. You just point out to him that he could make his weight more like that of other children, rather than pointing to his belly-button and how fat he is around there.

You show him the numbers—so many pounds gained in the last year and how, if he gained less, he would really be able to look just the way he would like to look. Which is like everybody else—although you don't have to point that out.

Most kids haven't even thought about wanting to look like others, or like anything in particular. But if you're telling a child that if he doesn't gain so much weight, then in a year or two years he will look the way he would like to look, he might think about how he really wants to look.

And it becomes an acceptable goal—because you are not putting him on a restrictive, weight-losing diet.

SUPPORTING THE EFFORT

Family support can be extremely important to a youngster embarked on weight control.

Obviously enough, his meals should be planned with his needs in mind. But in fact he should not be eating meals that are greatly different from those of the rest of the family, even if his plate may have a different balance and emphasis, such as more of fiber and less of fat than anyone else's.

Actually, the chances are that other members of the family, including one or both parents, could benefit from the same regimen—and in the process, help the child.

Many overweight children have overweight parents and siblings. Undesirable eating habits are rarely seen in just one child in a family.

And remember that what we are talking about all through this book is not a restrictive reducing diet but rather the development of sound eating patterns and habits that bring weight under control.

That could be appropriate for almost all American families —and certainly for most, if not all, families in which overweight is really a more or less general problem, even if most pronounced in a particular child.

Our attitudes as adults toward food have great bearing on the attitudes of our children. Children don't go so much by what we say as by what we do. The parent who tells a child to cut down on high-calorie snacks or other foods while he himself is unwrapping a calorie-loaded candy bar is giving the child mixed messages.

It's somewhat like the experience I had as a fat child, not with my family but when I was taken for a medical checkup, and the doctor, who proved to be a grotesquely fat man, duly examined me and then announced that *I* was fat and had to lose weight. And I said to my mother later, "How can that fat pig tell me that I have to lose weight!"

There is some tendency to think that adults have to live by different standards from those for children—that while you can enforce something on a child, you can't enforce on an adult because the adult has lived with a bad habit for too long and doesn't have the strength to give it up.

But that is "sticking" it to a kid.

Youngsters get their strength from adults; they get their control from adults. Through most of childhood, until they are old enough to make most decisions on their own and can be trusted to handle decisions on their own, they depend on us to control them.

If there is a constant war between parent and child for control, it is not a war the child really wants to win. He may want to win a battle here and there because he thinks that this or that is very important to him. But no child is really happy if he feels that his parents are not in control.

A parent who can't control himself is not likely to be able to control his child. And a parent who is willing to sit in front of his child and consume food that he tells his child not to consume is giving the child several messages.

One is "You have to do this, but I will not. It's okay for me to be fat." Well, the child just cannot understand that.

Another is "You are expected to be in control, but I can't control myself." And that is something no child can swallow. To a child, a parent is strong; the child is not. He, the child,

cannot be expected to have strength to accomplish something
if his parent cannot accomplish it.

GOOD FOR THE CHILD . . .
GOOD FOR THE FAMILY

As we have noted repeatedly, when we talk in this book
about the diet the overweight child should be on, we are talking about his or her learning to eat what he or she needs to
eat to be the right weight. We are not talking about losing
weight.

It stands to reason that what a child needs to eat to be the
right weight is, at once, a good diet for him—and for everyone
in the family.

Of course, other members of the family—depending upon
age, size, physical activity, and other factors—may need to
eat more or less than the overweight child.

But if, aside from any differences in quantities, everyone in
the family adopts the same patterns of eating—nutritious,
healthy, weight-controlling patterns—then the child is living
in an environment no longer hostile to him and his way of
eating.

To suggest that this may be punishing family members who
are not overweight is very much to miss the point.

If, indeed, you think punishment is involved, you will almost certainly convey that idea to your child. And why should
a fat child accept the idea of being punished for being fat?

But eating properly, eating to get all needed nourishment
and promote health while at the same time keeping control of
weight, is anything but punishment.

It's what all of us need—and it is really never too late to
make it an accomplishable goal. That can make you, as a
parent, feel good about yourself, and good too about contributing in a very major way to your youngster's health and hap-
piness.

12
Diet Pills

Forget all else. Unquestionably, for millions, the best of all wonder drugs would have to be one that simply melted away fat, that allowed effortless weight control.

It doesn't exist—nor is it likely to. But there is certainly no shortage of drugs marketed as weight-control aids.

In terms of adult use of such aids, the *Medical Letter*, a highly regarded publication for physicians, has observed: "There is no good evidence that phenylpropanolamine, oral benzocaine, or any other drug can help obese patients achieve long-term weight reduction. The only satisfactory treatment for obesity is a life-long change in patterns of food intake and physical activity."

And for children—for more, even, than those sufficient reasons—I believe strongly that diet pills should not be used.

AMPHETAMINES

In midsummer 1981, the Governor of the State of New York signed a bill making it illegal for any physician to prescribe amphetamines for the purpose of helping a patient lose or control weight. And the Medical Society of the State of New York, which normally resists restrictions on doctors' freedom to prescribe as they see fit, did not oppose the bill. It is consistent with the Society's formal opposition to amphetamine use for weight control.

93

Amphetamines are stimulants which act on the central nervous system. They do reduce appetite, but tolerance to this effect develops within two to three weeks. Increasing the dose to regain the effect is dangerous; amphetamines can be addictive.

Moreover, the appetite-suppressing effect of amphetamines is inseparable from their stimulating effect, which can cause insomnia. This limits the drugs' usefulness in the evening, when much overeating occurs.

And additionally, amphetamines have other undesirable side effects. They may elevate blood pressure and may cause palpitations, nervousness, irritability, dizziness, and upset stomach.

PHENYLPROPANOLAMINE

Related to the amphetamines, phenylpropanolamine has long been widely used as a nasal decongestant, both alone and in combination cold remedies.

It is now available, too, in many over-the-counter "appetite suppressants" such as Dexatrim, Prolamine, Spantrol, Appedrine, Bio Slim, Dietac, and P.V.M.

Is the drug effective? So some believe. Yet as the *Medical Letter* has noted, in one published study of 66 obese patients, the greatest weight loss was achieved not by anyone on phenylpropanolamine but by someone who, for comparison purposes, had been given a placebo, or look-alike–but–inert preparation.

Like amphetamines, phenylpropanolamine may cause nervousness, dizziness, and sleeplessness. Other possible undesirable effects include rapid pulse, palpitations, nausea, and nasal dryness.

Physicians are concerned that the drug is available without prescription. The drug companies themselves note that it should not be taken by anyone with heart disease, high blood pressure, diabetes, or thyroid or other disease—all conditions that may afflict the overweight, often without their awareness. And the companies also advise against use of phenylpropanolamine by anyone under the age of 18 except possibly with the advice of a physician.

OTHER AMPHETAMINELIKE AGENTS

Physicians can prescribe a number of other appetite-suppressant drugs such as diethylpropion and phentermine, almost all of them derivatives of amphetamines.

As with amphetamines, tolerance develops in a few weeks, so they lose effectiveness unless potentially dangerous larger doses are taken. They can be habit-forming. And among their adverse effects may be blood-pressure elevation, restlessness, insomnia, tremor, headache, hives, and palpitations.

Recently, when the U.S. Food and Drug Administration reviewed some 200 medical studies of amphetaminelike agents, it found that drug treatment produced only an extra half-pound of weight loss a week. As some authorities have pointed out, since tolerance develops within a few weeks and drug makers suggest discontinuing treatment at that point rather than increasing the dose, the average added benefit from appetite suppressants is only in the range of 1 to 2 pounds of weight loss—hardly worth the risks.

BULK PRODUCERS

Another type of over-the-counter appetite suppressant contains carboxymethylcellulose, which provides bulk to help satisfy the feeling of hunger caused by emptiness.

But one can accomplish the same result, quite naturally and healthily, without pills simply by eating high-fiber, low-calorie vegetables.

DIURETICS ("WATER PILLS")

These prescription drugs are not appetite suppressants and do not help rid the body of excess fat. Without any effect on fat deposits, they only promote excretion of water, and the water is replaced promptly when drug use is stopped.

Actually, most dieters lose excess water when they start dieting without using diuretics. This accounts for the early rapid weight loss many dieters experience.

Used indiscriminately, diuretics can upset the body's normal mineral balance, leading to potentially serious losses of sodium and potassium. They may produce nausea, weakness, and dizziness.

THYROID COMPOUNDS

These speed up metabolism—the body's handling of foods —and may bring about some loss of weight. But except for someone who actually needs a thyroid preparation because of low thyroid-gland functioning, thyroid compounds can upset the body's entire hormone balance. In the person with a normally functioning thyroid gland, they can produce hyperthyroidism, with such symptoms as irritability, abnormal heart rhythms, and possible heart failure.

THE ANESTHETIC

Benzocaine, a local anesthetic agent sometimes used to soothe skin irritations, itching, and burning and included in some throat lozenges, sprays, and cough syrups, is also an ingredient in some over-the-counter appetite suppressants and can be found too in special chewing gums or candies. It is supposed to dull the taste buds and discourage eating. But there are no adequate studies demonstrating effectiveness.

PILLS FOR CHILDREN

I think the usefulness of diet pills in adults is limited at best to the beginning of dieting as an aid in getting started. They cannot be depended on over a long period of time for weight control. Moreover, a loss of appetite without a proper diet plan may result in the eating of a less balanced diet without achieving the desired effect on weight.

Considering their limited usefulness and their potential side effects and dangers, I firmly believe that diet pills should not be used by children.

There is an additional very real philosophical consideration when it comes to the use of diet pills for children. And that is that our young people should not be led to believe that pills can lead to simple solutions for complex problems. Obesity is a particularly complex and emotionally charged problem in the older child and adolescent who is trying to deal with a constantly changing self-image and who is grappling with issues of self-control.

13
Camps for
Overweight Children

Camps for overweight children have become a burgeoning industry. In addition to individually owned weight-loss camps which are prospering, there are chains of diet camps for youngsters being advertised from coast to coast. There are camps for girls, camps for boys, and camps for boys and girls together.

In the course of writing this book, I checked on a number of the camps and can make this report on what, generally, their strengths are, what their weaknesses may be, and where they may fit into the overall effort to help an overweight child overcome his or her problem.

THE PROGRAMS AND COSTS

Youngsters' "fat camps," as they are sometimes called, do tend to be expensive, and that may be a major consideration for many parents.

Prices range, as of this writing, between $1,500 and $2,500 for 4- to 8-week sessions. The least expensive program was $900 for a 3-week session.

It should be noted that with proper documentation, some or all of the cost may be tax-deductible as a medical expense.

The aim of all the camps is weight reduction. Some emphasize that more than others. For example, one camp for boys aged 8 to 18 advertises "LOSE 20–50 POUNDS." Another, in a newspaper feature story, boasts of its 358 boys and girls going home and leaving behind a total of 8,000 pounds—an average of more than 22 pounds each.

All the camps checked are under the supervision of a physician or dietitian. They use calorie-restricted diets—commonly in the range of 1,100 to 1,300 calories. That does not constitute severe restriction for a child. And the diets are well rounded, though not individualized.

Lodgings are excellent. And the camps provide a striking array of facilities for sports and other activities.

As an example, the facilities at one camp include football and soccer fields, softball diamonds, indoor and outdoor basketball courts, a lake, a heated swimming pool, a sauna, a horse and riding ring, a quarter-mile track, an archery range, a circuit course, wrestling and tumbling mats, biking and hiking trails, street-hockey courts, a handball court, tennis courts, a golf course, a karate hall, volleyball courts, and tetherball courts.

POTENTIAL BENEFITS

Enforcing a calorie-restricted diet is, of course, simplified to some extent in a camp because of the unavailability of food except at mealtimes. As youngsters are told at one camp: "If you must have a Big Mac—well, you'll have to hike eighteen miles round trip, up and down hills, to get it."

With all the kids in a fat camp in the same boat—overweight —there is opportunity for group support in attempting to achieve a common objective.

And the almost constant activities can be very influential in moderating a child's urge to eat.

There is plenty of opportunity for exercise. Moreover, the fact that all the children in camp are overweight encourages many who have previously withdrawn from all sports to come out and play and benefit. None of the taunting about being fat that often stops obese kids from participating in activities that could help them reduce is there. Anyone who calls anyone else fat can expect to have the same taunt thrown right back.

Many of the camps provide nutritional counseling and follow-up programs, so that if children do learn their lessons about eating and get involved in follow-up, there is a chance they may learn to make permanent changes in their eating habits. Some of the camps mail newsletters which, for example, may report that this or that camper has lost so many more pounds; another has begun an athletic career. Some mail diet menus and snack suggestions, portion-control and exercise programs. Some offer 10-month cassette follow-up and maintenance programs including diet and exercise information.

A POTENTIAL FOR FAILURE?

There is, of course, no guarantee that weight loss achieved in camp will be maintained.

The potential for failure lies in the return of a child to an environment at home that is likely to be markedly different from the camp environment. At home, there is none of the same provision for keeping busy constantly with many activities. And family eating habits may be very different from those learned at camp—and in fact, are likely to be, or there would probably have been no need for camp in the first place.

In these circumstances, it can be difficult if not impossible for a child who may have lost a considerable amount of weight during the weeks in camp to maintain the loss.

What may contribute to the difficulty, too, is the fact that in camp the child has been on a calorie-restricted weight-loss diet and hasn't really had an opportunity to learn to eat in a way that maintains weight. And if, upon returning home, faced with a household full of food, the child fails to maintain loss and begins to gain weight, discouragement may set in. And discouragement is one of the main causes of failure for dieters.

SHOULD YOUR CHILD GO? SOME GUIDELINES

The decision as to whether a child should go to a weight-loss camp must, of course, be a very personal one.

For one thing, whether a child can benefit from a camp program will depend on his or her feelings about camping. Some children don't like to go to camp; some very much look forward to the opportunity to be with and join in activities with other children of their age.

I am sure that there are overweight children who dread the idea of going to a regular camp because they feel that they can't fit in, can't play games well, are unable to compete against normal-weight youngsters. They might love the idea of going to a "fat" camp if they could just get over the idea it is a fat camp—if the prospect were presented to them as an opportunity to be with people who have similar problems or people who have the same athletic abilities and interests and with whom they can have a good time.

Is a fat camp essential for an overweight child? Hardly. It can be a useful adjunct, but it is certainly not the sine qua non of effective weight control.

I have no compelling reason to discourage parents from using weight-loss camps. I do have a reservation. I do not fully agree with the idea of having a child lose weight, particularly large amounts of weight, because of the potential for regaining the weight, since when you lose weight, you can't really learn how to maintain weight. And I would much prefer it if the aim of a camp were not to produce weight loss but simply to offer youngsters a program of activities with their peers along with nutritional information to help them learn how to eat properly, without emphasis on weight loss.

If you as a parent decide that you would like to send your child to camp, undoubtedly he or she can gain something from the experience. I would caution, however, that any weight loss achieved will not be maintained unless you are prepared to follow through with any necessary changes in family meals and eating patterns and with effort on your part to encourage more regular physical activity on the child's part.

14
Special Considerations:
Feeding the Baby

Today, many hundreds of thousands of children are over-weight. Many, even most, of them will grow up having to fight fat.

In some cases, of course, genetic factors may be involved. Just what those factors are is not as yet clear. There is some evidence that body build may play a role. Possibly account-able sometimes may be an inherited misfunctioning of the center in the brain that regulates appetite or a fault in the body system that determines how food is used.

But recent research suggests that most people who become obese start out with normal body chemistry and controls which may become disturbed by a weight gain.

Certainly, feeding is an important part of an infant's life. And it is likely that feeding habits and attitudes, and perhaps unconscious feelings about food which develop in infancy, will affect a person for the rest of his life.

Overfeeding—for any reason—during infancy may set the stage for childhood and adult obesity.

Overfeeding occurs when parents encourage plumpness out of a mistaken idea that the fatter the baby, the healthier, or when they equate plentiful feeding with caring and good par-enting, or when they feed to relieve fussiness or boredom or to encourage sleep.

It may be hard to refuse a crying baby who wants a bottle or a cookie, but it is no harder and no less important than teaching children how we expect them to behave regarding other matters, and it is in their best interest. It does not become easier to restrict a child's eating and change his eating habits when he is 6 years old if he has been overeating all his short life.

Adults determine what little children eat and when they eat. A baby can be trim only if someone feeds him properly. And he can be fat only if someone overfeeds him.

THE PERSISTING MYTH

A few years ago, in a study of 130 infants, Johns Hopkins University pediatricians made a disturbing discovery.

It's a fact that the needs of a 2-month-old infant can be met adequately through formula or breast milk alone. Yet 93 percent of the infants of that age in the study were being fed dry cereal as well, and 70 percent were also receiving strained fruit.

The total caloric intake was about 30 percent above recommended allowances. And the pattern remained the same—feeding to excess—when the babies were studied again at the age of 7 months.

A basic problem, the investigators reported, remains the false notion of many people that a fat baby is healthier than a skinny one.

A recent New York City Department of Health study turned up the finding that it is not the baby but the mother who molds the baby's appetite. Rather than listen to medical advice about sensible diets, the surveyed mothers acknowledged that they paid more attention to advice from relatives, to TV commercials, and even to old wives' tales.

Many authorities see at work a spirit of keeping up with the Joneses by having an infant gobble up formula in order to produce a better-looking growth chart—a decidedly unhealthy spirit. One obesity specialist looks upon the digestive tract as "the biggest battleground between mother and child in early childhood" and believes it is going to take a Herculean effort to encourage mothers to nourish children sensibly and not excessively if millions are to be saved from a lifetime of obesity.

THE FAT-CELL PHENOMENON

One theory—accepted by many but not all investigators—proposes at least one reason why it is important not to overfeed in early childhood and why possibly such overfeeding can lead to lifelong weight difficulty.

It has to do with fat cells—tiny structures which all of us have located throughout the body, common in tissue between skin and muscles, with large concentrations in the abdomen and around such organs as the kidneys and heart.

They act to collect and hold fat from food, storing it for delivery into the bloodstream and burning as energy when needed.

It is not known whether we all, at birth, have the same number of fat cells. It is known that once a fat cell appears in the body, it remains for a lifetime although the amount of fat stored in any given cell can vary from day to day and year to year.

And it also appears that the number of fat cells can multiply in the first months of life, tripling or even quadrupling.

According to the theory, such multiplication of fat cells presents a considerable problem. The baby who is fed in a way that produces no such multiplication will have far less trouble with obesity throughout a lifetime than the infant fed in excess and left thereafter with an excess of fat cells.

For the cells, it is hypothesized, do not just sit there quietly. Some investigators believe that the fat cells may communicate with the appetite center in the brain, sending messages of a need to be filled and so leading to excessive appetite.

REASONABLE FEEDING

Infant-feeding recommendations have changed considerably in recent years, even just the past half-dozen years.

Babies often used to start solids at 4 weeks of age. They were switched from formula to low-fat or skim milk at 3 months. Today, we recommend formula for 9 to 12 months. Skim milk is not recommended because of its high protein and solute load. We avoid introducing solids until a baby is at least 4 months old.

104

I recommend what I call a modified demand-feeding schedule. If it is less than 2 hours since a feeding, I consider that a baby generally does not need to be fed. If it is much after 3 hours and a baby is fussy, chances are he needs to be fed. One should not be a clock watcher, but when it is not feeding time one should not immediately offer a fussy baby a bottle. There are many things one can try with a crying baby before feeding him.

The bottle can be a problem in the toddler who uses it as a pacifier. Bottles should be offered to older babies only at mealtimes. Toddlers should not spend the day walking around with their bottles.

SOLID FOODS: NO RUSH—
AND GOOD REASON WHY NOT

There has been a tendency for mothers to want to feed their babies solids as early as possible. The tendency, which continues, was even encouraged by some physicians until relatively recently.

I can remember that when my firstborn was a month old and we started him on cereal—I was a medical student at the time—my father-in-law was a happy man. "Now that the baby is *eating*," he observed, "he is at least half a man."

That was a common attitude then. It carries over to this day. I see many mothers in my office who are very anxious to have their babies start solid foods. They are especially so if the baby is not sleeping through the night or appears to be what they think is hungry. Many tell me of other mothers whose babies have stopped crying and are sleeping through the night because they started solid foods. But I believe that that is largely coincidence; a baby starts sleeping through the night when he is ready to. Most babies do so between 4 and 6 weeks, some not until later. And we have experience with many mothers who have not introduced solids until 4 to 6 months and whose babies started to sleep through long before then. And the babies have grown well, too.

A major reason I prefer not to start solid foods early is that in a baby under 4 months of age, the swallowing mechanism is immature.

When you put solid food into the mouth of a child under 4

months of age, all he can do is move his tongue back and forth, and some of the food goes down while some comes out. And you take what is on the child's chin and shove it back in, and eventually the food goes down.

The baby may be full as you keep shoving the food in—and the food keeps going in and eventually going down because the baby has no control until he is at least 4 months old.

If you give a baby a bottle and he gets full, he simply stops sucking. If you're nursing and the baby is full, he pulls away from the breast.

But until 4 months, a baby is not able to stop taking solid foods, and you can be literally stuffing him the way you stuff the goose for Christmas.

There are two potential carry-overs.

One is that the baby may learn to ignore the sensation of satiation if he is constantly being overfed.

The other, if you believe in the fat-cell theory, is that you are already laying down excess fat cells to be carried for life.

Another factor may enter the picture. Many babies, unable to handle solid foods well, become irritable when fed them. Instead of realizing the child doesn't want the solids, Mother may take that as a challenge. She may then adopt the tactic of giving the baby a nipple to suck on, then pulling it out and shoving solids in.

The child may even get angry. Normally, if a baby screams hysterically about something you are doing, you would stop. But many mothers who initiate early solid feeding and realize that the baby isn't doing well with it presume the baby is screaming because he is not being satisfied fast enough. And so they keep shoving the stuff down.

Actually, when a Committee on Nutrition of the American Academy of Pediatrics reviewed the history of the use of solid foods, it found that solid or supplemental foods were seldom offered to infants before 1 year of age until about 1920. Breast milk, for the most part, or modified cow's-milk formulas supplied all or most of the nutritional needs of infants during the first year. The first supplements to the diet were cod-liver oil to prevent rickets and orange juice to prevent scurvy.

Over the next half-century, there were recommendations that some cereals and strained vegetables and fruits be given

to babies at about 6 months of age in order to supply iron, vitamins, and possibly other factors, and to help prepare the infant for a more diversified diet.

But then, as the Academy has noted in a recent report, "A much wider variety of infant foods became available, and these were introduced into the infant's diet earlier and earlier. Some of the reasons for earlier introduction of solid foods were the desire of mothers to see their infants gain weight rapidly, the ready availability of convenient forms of solid foods, and the mistaken assumption that added solid foods help the infant to sleep through the night."

And in that report, the Academy's Committee on Nutrition went on to take note of the possible role of early introduction of solid foods in obesity and to make recommendations.

Supplemental foods, it pointed out,

should be introduced when the infant is able to sit with support and has good neuromuscular control of the head and neck. At this stage of development, the infant will be able to indicate a desire for food by opening his mouth and leaning forward, and to indicate [lack of] interest or satiety by leaning back and turning his head away.

At this time, about 4 to 6 months of age, a variety of foods should be introduced one at a time, at intervals of a week or more. The sequence of foods is not critical, but iron-fortified, single-grain infant cereals are a good early choice.

The addition of individual (not mixed) vegetables, fruits, or meats introduces a variety of foods and sets the pattern for a diversified diet.

With the background of these guidelines for infants as a group, the age of introduction of supplemental foods for individual infants cannot be set rigidly; rather, it depends on rate of growth, stage of development, and level of activity.

On the basis of present knowledge, no nutritional advantage results from the introduction of supplemental foods prior to 4 to 6 months of age. This conclusion is essentially the same as in the Committee statement of 1958, but it deserves reemphasis because of the continuing widespread and possibly harmful effects of introducing supplemental foods at 1 or 2 months of age, or earlier.

15
Special Considerations:
But Is Your Child
Really Underweight?

It's surprising how many parents become extraordinarily—and almost always unnecessarily—concerned about a child who, to them, appears to be underweight, much too thin, needing to eat more.

I had a 5-year-old in my office recently. He had several problems, none easily solvable but none very serious, among them bed-wetting and soiling. Nor was he an overwhelmingly bright child. But if nothing else, his growth was entirely normal.

Yet a main concern of his father's, even in the face of the real problems, was "How can I make this child fatter? He is so skinny!"

I showed the father where the child's height and weight fell on the growth chart. Weight was right for height, and both were within normal range.

But the father was not at all impressed by that bit of information. He looked at his child again. "Too skinny," he said.

I asked him why he was so concerned, what did he think was going to happen. "Any child so skinny," he said, "just can't be healthy."

We have two misconceptions there.

The first was that the child was skinny. The father was seeing in his youngster what a perfectly normal child of that age looks like and still was convinced he was much below normal, a skinny lad.

And his second idea was no less a misconception: that you can't be healthy if you are, in fact, skinny.

What happens to be true—except in the case of a child who is malnourished either because of unavailability of food or because of an illness that prevents normal weight gain and growth—is that skinny children are at least as healthy as children of normal weight and undoubtedly healthier than children who are overweight.

If I had to make a choice for my children between over- and underweight, with no middle ground allowed, I would pick underweight anytime. And I would have no worries about it.

Now, of course, if a child is underweight and if there has never been any assurance for the parents that nonetheless all is well, if the child has not been examined by a physician, then he should be. But if you know your child is healthy, that there is no illness causing him to be underweight, there is no reason for concern.

Actually, many parents have a false perception of skinniness in a child, and often it stems from lack of awareness of some of the details of how children grow.

THE WAY THEY SPROUT

At birth, most babies today weigh between 6 and 10 pounds. And by 6 months they usually double their birth weight.

Then there is some slowing of growth. In the next 6 months, babies put on an amount equal to what they did in their first 6 months—but that, of course, is not a doubling of weight.

The growth rate between 1 and 2 years slows down further. If you look at the growth charts elsewhere in this book, you can see the curve for weight flattening.

For children between ages 2 and 7 years, the growth rate slows even further. These children are not growing less because they are eating less; they are eating less because they are growing less.

Children between 2 and 7 may eat less for a variety of reasons. But one of the most important reasons they don't have as big an appetite as you might expect is the slowing of their growth rate. Their requirements for growth are so low that in fact they sometimes may eat less than what they did even as babies.

Appearances can be deceiving as children grow.

Babies between 1 and 2 years of age—toddlers beginning to walk around—have a significant amount of baby fat, and the fat is distributed in different fashion from the fat of older children.

They tend to have more fat around the legs, but nothing very impressive in the buttocks. Look at the rear ends of babies with fat legs and there is practically nothing there. They don't develop any significant amount of musculature in the buttocks until after they have been walking about for some time. But they have a significant amount of fat around the middle, and many have double chins. And that can be normal for babies who are not overweight.

But then the fat distribution begins to change—so much so that by age 3 a child who still is in the same weight percentile he was in at age 1 looks skinnier. His body is slimmer; he is taller; his legs are no longer fat; his face is no longer fat; his middle is no longer fat. He has developed more muscles in legs and buttocks and has strong musculature in his abdomen so that everything doesn't hang out. And he will look skinnier to you even if he hasn't lost weight.

THE PARENTAL ANXIETY STARTS

Go back for a moment to the child between years 1 and 2 when his appetite is already slowing down. He is also coming off baby food. Baby food has a high concentration of water; water, in fact, is one of the main ingredients. Necessarily. Until the child's swallowing mechanism fully matures and he can handle solid food well, water has to be added.

So whether she realizes it or not, a mother gives a child a larger volume of baby food than she would of nonpureed solid food for the same amount of nutrition because with baby food she is giving the baby a lot of water.

And so when a child starts eating more solid foods, with

much less water in them, he may not want the same volume he took when eating pureed baby foods.

And now, too, he is striking out for independence: he wants to feed himself.

Add, too, that at this point he is developing other interests besides eating. Eating is no longer virtually the whole of his life; he is paying attention to what is going on around him.

We all remember when our infants would wake up and often the only reason was that they were screaming to eat. Well, now our 2-year-old spends a lot of time awake. Eating is not the most important thing in his life. He may get cranky when he is hungry, but he doesn't necessarily start screaming for food. If there is something he wants to do in the midst of eating, he will eat just enough to satisfy himself and then get on to doing what he wants. Other interests have become more central in his life.

And what with the child's less intense preoccupation with eating, and his striking out for independence and increasing insistence on feeding himself, Mother may wonder: Will this child get enough to eat?

And when all of that is coupled, too, with the child's decreased need for food with slowing growth rate and his apparent change in body habitus, it is all too easy for Mother to become overwhelmingly anxious that her child is wasting away before her eyes because he will not let her feed him good, nutritious foods.

And that is when feeding problems may begin.

Mother starts pushing the child to eat; the child may resist; and the fights begin.

But some children who are more passive and who feel it is important to please Mommy will sit and have the food shoved into them. And that may put them on the road to obesity.

At this point, too, we may see the "clean-plate syndrome" developing.

Mother, in her desire to make sure her child eats, will teach him that he must clean his plate, finish everything on it. And in so doing, she teaches him something he will carry with him for the rest of his life.

There is only one good, day-in–day-out reason for the normal person to eat: because of hunger. And those of us who carry with us guilt that there are starving people in the world and the belief that we must therefore eat everything on our plates have been saddled with something totally wrong.

Can we really be said to help the starving when we ourselves get fat?

CHANGES WITH THE YEARS

The fact is that most children between ages 2 and 7 who appear skinny and cause concern to their mothers not only are normal and healthy but are eating what is right for them.

And if Mother can get over any initial panic that she may be doing a bad job as a mother because her child looks so skinny, she will discover that between ages 7 and 10 the child's appetite will pick up because his growth rate begins to pick up.

And then between ages 10 and 13, with the onset of pre-puberty and early adolescence, growth rate and appetite will pick up even more. And then, as a growth spurt occurs in mid- to late puberty, the child's appetite will become extraordinary and Mother may well complain that he is eating her out of house and home.

Most adolescents will be starting their growth spurt between ages 13 and 15 and will be in the throes of the major spurt between 15 and 17. Then they will begin to slow down. But many boys will continue to grow in height until 20 or 21, although most girls will have reached their adult height between 16 and 18.

These children, along with their naturally increased appetites, may also carry the burden of parental attitudes. Those who were told throughout their early childhood that they were too skinny and had to finish everything on the plate and who may have been encouraged to eat a lot of "goodies"—perhaps ice cream and other sweets—may well first become obese during adolescence if they haven't become so during childhood.

16
Special Considerations: Anorexia Nervosa

She is a 16-year-old, attractive, of normal weight, an excellent student. Suddenly, she goes on a diet and loses weight—excessively. She claims she cannot eat with her family. She complains of feeling fat and ugly. She keeps dieting to the point of emaciation.

When her parents finally succeed in getting her to a physician, a complete physical examination and workup rule out any malignancy or gastrointestinal disorder. The final diagnosis: anorexia nervosa.

The disease recently has become a popular subject for newspaper and magazine articles and for television programs.

And any parent with an adolescent daughter who is either dieting or planning to diet may be seriously concerned about the possibility of anorexia nervosa.

I think it is important to emphasize here at once that dieting to the point of emaciation is certainly an aspect of anorexia nervosa—but *dieting is not the cause of anorexia nervosa.*

And I think it important to emphasize here too that if anything, the kind of weight control we are talking about in this book is more likely to be a helpful safeguard against rather than precipitant of anorexia nervosa.

It can, occasionally, affect a boy—but only very occasionally. It is primarily seen in adolescent girls and young adult women, mostly in the age range of 12 to 25.

Anorexia nervosa was first described about a century ago and for long was considered extremely rare. In the past decade, however, there has been a marked apparent increase in incidence. Some researchers currently estimate that anorexia nervosa is now so prevalent that 1 of every 250 girls between the ages of 12 and 18 suffers from it and 1 or 2 girls in every high school may have it.

There are suspicions among some researchers that the attention the disorder has been getting in the media may be inspiring what one child and adolescent psychiatrist calls "a mass hysteria in which anorexic girls are becoming an idol of other adolescent girls."

Anorexic girls lose at least 25 percent of body weight, and the loss may even range up to 50 percent. They lose weight by cutting back drastically on food intake or by eating only foods low in fat or carbohydrates. Many at times induce vomiting or take laxatives, diuretics ("water pills"), or enemas to rid themselves of food and liquids. Many overexercise, spending hours a day at it.

Along with weight loss, anorexics develop a low body temperature, a decreased pulse rate, and often a drop in blood pressure. Many stop having their menstrual periods. There may be edema, or fluid swellings, especially in the ankles and legs. Lanugo—newbornlike hair—may appear on the skin.

Clearly, anorexia is a psychiatric disorder. Its victims experience a severely distorted body image. Standing in front of a mirror, viewing themselves, seeing little more than skin and bones, they refuse to consider that they are underweight, persist in the idea that they are grossly obese and have to lose weight.

Many lose their appetite for food completely—but many go on binges of eating, known as bulimic episodes, during which they gorge themselves far beyond the point any normal person would consider, then often follow this by vomiting everything up.

WHAT CAUSES ANOREXIA?

There are, as yet, no final, definitive answers. There are many observations and theories about possible causes.

Some investigators believe that a primary factor may be a desperate struggle for control and a sense of identity. Dr. Hilde Bruch, a distinguished authority on anorexia and author of *The Golden Cage* and *Eating Disorders*, has observed: "Girls with conforming personalities feel obliged to do something that demands a great degree of independence in order to be respected and recognized. When they get stuck, the only independence they feel they have is to control their own bodies."

Some investigators believe that many anorexics fear growing up and facing responsibilities and use anorexia as a means to stop the process. "Some," remarks Dr. Meir Gross, head of the section of child and adolescent psychiatry at the Cleveland Clinic in Cleveland, Ohio, "have a delayed psychosexual development and cannot cope with the transition through adolescence. Their interest in sex is decreased, and few anorexic patients are interested in dating or getting married during the course of the illness."

Some psychiatrists who have looked into family structure for causes believe that anorexia may be used as a means of manipulating or punishing a neglectful or domineering mother. And what, indeed, they note, could be a more effective attention-getting device than starvation!

Many anorexics, in my experience, do have disturbed family relationships. Some were overweight to begin with and their mothers felt they should lose weight. And many of these girls, although you can't get them to eat in the presence of their parents, we can turn around once they are hospitalized by slowly introducing feeding and not pushing the matter until gradually their tolerance for food increases.

But many persist in the gross misconception that they are extraordinarily fat even though they are severely underweight.

Actually, many anorexic girls were only slightly overweight to begin with. Their idea in going on a diet was to lose weight and then make friends and become popular.

Their primary problem was never obesity. Their difficulty in getting along with other people was part of their difficulty in getting along with their families and part of their difficulties in coping with life.

And they started out with a distorted self-image—of being fat and ugly, unloved and unlovable. Because of that ingrained self-image and because of their psychiatric problems, they are unable to see that they are losing weight, unable to develop a feeling of success over becoming the way they want to be. They still do not feel lovable and do not go out seeking to establish normal relationships with people.

I've observed, as you may have too, that many overweight people who have been on a weight-reducing diet, particularly one that brought quick loss, have difficulty in adapting to the idea that they are no longer fat. But they don't have such a distorted self-image that they take their dieting to the point of emaciation and still consider themselves overweight.

Anorexics, starving themselves, can become extraordinarily ill. Some are so protein-malnourished that when they start eating again their bodies become swollen because their bloodstream lacks enough protein to hold fluid normally. They have lost more than fat; they have lost muscle mass. Their organs do not function properly because in the face of such severe protein malnutrition, they use up not only fat but also many of the body cells. They are literally living off their bodies.

I recall some hospitalized anorexic cases that hit me hard when I was in my residency. The youngest was 11. When I first met her, she was extremely thin, with a very hollow face and big staring eyes—the kind of thing you see in pictures from concentration camps.

She was adamant: "You will not make me eat. I cannot be made to eat." And she was not impressed with the idea that she might die. As far as she was concerned, we could save her from dying if it came to that. If she was nearing death, she would be willing to let us put in an intravenous line and give her some fluids. And we replenished her fluids a few times that way when she was getting near the edge. But she was absolutely adamant about not being tube-fed; she would take no food. She was not very communicative, and anything she did say centered on the one idea: nobody could force her to eat, including the doctors.

There was also the 22-year-old young lady who was extraordinarily vivacious and who would go to extremes, one moment saying how fat she was and how much she had to lose weight, but then, while walking around with no clothes on her pathetically skinny body except a bathrobe, she would, the next moment, open the robe to other people and say, "Look how beautiful I am." She was very bizarre. And even though she was 22, she clearly had a disturbed relationship with her family, and many of the fights about eating occurred when her family was visiting her in the hospital.

Now, I hope it is clear that when I talk about a disturbed relationship with the family, I don't mean to cast blame on any one person. The relationship is disturbed—and the relationship involves interaction between people. It is not a one-sided matter.

TREATMENT

There is no one approach to what may be the best treatment for anorexia nervosa. But there is agreement that malnutrition is the first concern and must be controlled before the psychological problems are dealt with.

Hospitalization is often essential. Very severe anorexics may have so little reserve, nothing for their bodies to fall back on, that they may tip from malnutrition to cardiac arrest in no time.

And so we have to slowly replenish them, and sometimes that takes the form of putting a large intravenous line into one of the deep veins inside the body that can take necessary concentrated solutions of nutrients.

Once they have thus been pulled back, in effect, from the brink, we have to work on a program of trying to get them to eat. The aim is not to feed them huge amounts and put a lot of weight on them right away—but mainly to get them to eat enough so they will survive. Then comes psychotherapy.

The success rate?

When patients can be gotten into psychotherapy, the success rate is considered pretty good. Pretty good means that many will recover completely and once they are over the throes of anorexia nervosa and have gained weight and developed normal body habitus again, they can go on to a normal life without developing anorexia again. Some may still have significant personality disturbances and would do well to continue in psychotherapy until those are worked out.

And when I say the success rate is pretty good, I don't want to mislead you, either. There are still some deaths from anorexia nervosa. It is an illness that can kill.

And may I repeat here again a very essential point for any reader of this book.

The kind of weight control we are talking about here—with its emphasis on avoiding quick-loss diets in favor of keeping weight in check so a child can grow healthily into what will be his or her proper weight—has no relationship to anorexia nervosa. Anyone willing to stick with such sound control is certainly not headed in the direction of anorexic illness.

17
Common Questions and Answers

Q. *Considering that it can take a long time—perhaps discouragingly long—for a child to grow into his ideal weight, wouldn't it be better for him to lose, say, 10 or 15 pounds quickly at first so he can feel he has accomplished something?*

A. Absolutely not. First, because of the potential for ill effects on health and growth from rapid weight loss. Nor is it likely a child will have greater success trying to lose weight rapidly. Even children successful in losing at first reach a plateau, no longer lose rapidly, and may become discouraged and begin to gain again. Moreover, should a child actually succeed on a rapid-loss diet, at some point he will need to go on a maintenance diet—exactly what we've been talking about in this book. It's something that has to be done for the rest of life and depends upon learning proper nutrition and eating the right number of calories to maintain weight. So rather than starting off with a bang, learning nothing about maintenance, and perhaps getting discouraged and failing altogether, we urge starting out with what amounts to a diet that will get you to—and then automatically maintain—the weight you want for the rest of your life.

Q. *I don't allow my children to eat junk foods. So how could they have become fat?*

A. Whether or not a child becomes overweight depends on

caloric intake versus caloric outgo. If he consumes more than he burns, the body stores the excess as fat. It's not surprising when a child who eats snacks and junk foods on top of a normal diet gains weight. But an excess of very good food can add weight too.

Q. *My child doesn't overeat anything, yet he's overweight. Why?*

A. That's a *seeming* fact that puzzles many parents. Often, it turns out they have an unrealistic idea of how much a child *should* eat. Commonly, children's appetites decrease during the growth slowdown period between ages 2 and 7 years. And actually, a child who, in his parents' view, eats well during that period may be eating much more than normal—which is why, to parental surprise, he becomes overweight. It's also a fact that some parents have an unrealistic idea of how much a child actually is eating—which is why we suggest keeping a log. A child may eat relatively little at meals yet consume sizable amounts of calories via snacks and beverages between meals.

Q. *What do I do if my child becomes sick while on a weight-control program? Should the diet be changed?*

A. The diet discussed in this book is sound and nutritious at almost any time. There is rarely reason to alter it during illness. The child in most cases can recover and be perfectly healthy again on this kind of diet. Diarrhea may require a few diet modifications. Then, milk and milk products are best avoided.

Q. *What's to be done when a child is sick and refuses to eat?*

A. By all means, avoid trying to get the child to eat with high-calorie and junk-food bribes. The child is following his body's natural dictates. If his stomach were up to handling food, his appetite wouldn't be impaired. I think the purpose of teaching children good nutrition is defeated if we try to handle nutrition differently when they're ill. If a child simply has no appetite, that should be respected. Generally, sick children do well if they drink adequate fluids. Appetite will return

120

when the illness is over and most children will make up for any caloric loss.

Q. *If a child doesn't finish his meal, should he be allowed dessert?*

A. Unless a child is still hungry after a meal, he should not have an additional course. Dessert can be saved for a snack. Certainly, dessert shouldn't be used as a reward for eating and to encourage children to "clean their plates." It's not wrong to give a child dessert if he hasn't eaten everything on his plate. When my own children say they're full, have eaten almost nothing at dinner, but ask for dessert, I tell them, "If you weren't hungry for dinner, you can't possibly be hungry for dessert." But I don't make an association between cleaning up their plates and being rewarded with dessert. And once they've eaten reasonable portions so I know they're not going to be living on desserts alone, I have no qualms about letting them have dessert even if food is left on their plates. Children, I believe, should have their appetites for various foods respected as long as they are not overindulging in one type to the exclusion of others.

Q. *Once children are on a weight-control program, isn't it risky to let them have ice cream or any other treat? If they get it one time, won't they wonder why not another time?*

A. Older children have no problem in understanding that some foods are what you live on and others are special treats not to be eaten all the time. Older children also can understand the relationship between weight and what's eaten. They may not be happy about the special nature of treats, but it's not difficult to explain to them. A younger child may not understand—but he knows he has to eat what is given. From the day children learn the word "cookie," for example, and then start asking for cookies, sometimes you give them cookies and sometimes you say no. Children may not understand why it's sometimes yes and sometimes no, but they learn from early on that that's the way it is and the one who decides is Mommy or Daddy.

Q. What can we do about visiting relatives who bring treats and ruin a child's diet?

A. Ruin? Not really. Weight gain is a slow matter. To add a pound, 3,500 extra calories have to be consumed. A child isn't likely to consume that much extra in a day or weekend no matter how extravagantly "treatful" visiting relatives are. Nor is it what one does in a day or a weekend that counts significantly, but rather what's done over months and years. To be sure, 300, 600, 800 extra calories in a day or two may seem like a lot; but it is the regular, routine 100 extra daily calories adding up to 36,500 in a year that really count. We should, of course, try to enlist relatives in not pushing treats on the children. But since we do allow youngsters treats on special occasions, we need not become unduly alarmed about occasional visitations and profferings by relatives. And it can be helpful to offer an explanation to youngsters—about how different people have different eating habits, and Mom and Dad have spent a lot of time trying to understand what's good for their family in view of the fact that their family tends to have weight problems. Grandpa, Grandma, Uncle and Auntie haven't taken the time to think that through because they haven't had to deal with the problem. And so we, in this family, can appreciate them for bringing us things, for thinking well of us, but we still have to know what is best for us.

Q. Our problem isn't just occasional diet-spoiling by a relative. With both my husband and me working, Grandma and an aunt take turns caring for our child and seem to be undermining our attempts at controlling his weight. What can we do?

A. This can be a difficult problem to deal with and may require an honest look at what the actual situation is. Are the caretaking relatives fully aware of what the child's needs are —and are they doing the undermining intentionally? For an answer, the mother has to sit down with the caretakers and go over what the child's diet should be. It may be beneficial to have the caretakers read this book for a better understanding. Some older relatives may have difficulty accepting the idea

122

that a child should weigh less than what he does because they grew up with the idea of fat's being the essence of health. If having them read this book fails to help, it may be important to enlist the aid of your physician to sit down with the care-takers and explain to them how our attitudes toward fat have changed and what the child actually does need for health.

Q. *Can't fat babies be expected to grow out of their fat?*

A. Some do, but the statistics are pretty grim. A significant proportion of fat babies turn into adults who are also fat. But even if a child can grow out of his baby fat, why let him suffer being fat? If he is fat, then either his eating habits or his exercise habits or both are not suitable for him. And the younger he is, the easier it will be for him to learn new habits. And the kind of new habits we suggest learning in this book are not painful. Certainly, they are not nearly as painful as growing up fat and being teased and taunted.

Q. *What can one do when a child refuses to eat vegetables?*

A. Vegetables can be important in weight control because, among other things, many are nonfattening fillers. However, if your child refuses to eat vegetables, it doesn't have to mean he can't control his weight. But you shouldn't be willing to fill the gap with extra portions of other kinds of food that will add to his weight. If there are one or two vegetables in the low-calorie group that he is willing to eat, have no qualms about offering them as often as possible. Often, children can be encouraged to eat vegetables when they're prepared in a vari-ety of ways. But in the end, if your child stubbornly refuses them, he can still follow the other nutritional advice offered earlier in this book to try to control his weight without eating vegetables.

Q. *I'd like my child to eat more vegetable snacks, less of other kinds—but it has been no go. Any suggestions?*

A. If you've simply asked whether he'd like such snacks and he has said "Naw" or the equivalent—and especially if he doesn't see his parents eating them—his refusal is not surpris-ing. Try eating vegetable snacks yourself and letting him see you do so—and then offering them to him, especially when he is really hungry. He may be surprised—and so may you—to find that he enjoys them. It may help, too, if you serve them in attractive ways—perhaps cut into varied shapes or served shish-kebab fashion, with different-colored vegetables alternating on toothpicks.

Q. *How can anyone deprive a child of a cookie?*

A. This is a common question. The answer is that there is no need to do that in order to control weight. But we have to draw the line someplace—and maybe that place for your child is at two cookies, or three or four. Whatever it is, if a child has to cut down, you do have to draw the line. But it's not a matter of deprivation. If you had a child who became ill after eating cookies, you wouldn't have any second thoughts about eliminating cookies. Obesity is subtle. It creeps up slowly. It's only at a certain point that you realize a child is fat—and at that point you have to do something to cut down. Obesity, though not as dramatic as violent illness, takes its toll. And just as no parent would worry about deprivation when it comes to keeping a child away from something that would make him ill, so too with the cookie that contributes to obesity.

Q. *What can we do about the Halloween problem?*

A. Halloween is an occasion children can enjoy, and I don't think an overweight child should be cut out of it. There should, I believe, be limits on Halloween for all children. It's not essential for any child to canvass his entire neighborhood for candy. He can dress up, join with his friends, canvass the homes of several people he knows. And when he comes home, his candy collection should be inspected and anything that might be "garbage" or tainted should be removed from the bag. Then he should be allowed to have the rest of the candy in small amounts, on an occasional basis—and that will not destroy his diet.

Q. *How can you make a child aware he needs to diet?*

A. You can keep eyes and ears open to the problems all

obese children have sooner or later. Any child who reaches public school, if he wasn't aware of being fat before then, becomes aware at that point because of association with peers who are not at all hesitant about pointing it out to him—and also because of the effect of his weight on his ability to participate in the things that nonfat children do. A child comes home crying because he has been teased . . . a child comes home upset because he has not been chosen for the team . . . a girl comes home distraught because she is not being asked out on dates—these are occasions when a sympathetic parent can effectively, in a nonjudgmental way, suggest a solution. Almost invariably, if parents keep their eyes and ears open to an overweight child's concerns, they will find opportunity to introduce the idea of doing something about weight.

Q. Can a child be so muscular that he only seems to be overweight?

A. Muscle does weigh more than fat, and a muscular child may weigh more than another child of the same height—but the muscular child is not likely to look fat. When it comes to a preadolescent child, however, there isn't likely to be much musculature, since muscular development requires hormonal activity which comes with puberty.

Q. Are there criteria other than growth charts for determining whether a child is or isn't overweight?

A. Appearance is important. If a child looks fat, he may well be. But since children are growing, I think it's important to consider not only what they look like now but what their weight trend is. If they are continuing to gain more in weight then in height, then something should be done. So even if a child is not significantly obese at the moment, he needs to relearn his eating habits and perhaps his exercise habits as well if he is gaining more weight than he should be gaining.

Q. Are there differences in the nutritional needs of boys and girls?

A. Not for prepubescent boys and girls. Their growth rates

125

are just about the same, and so are their needs, for both calories and nutrients. Later, with puberty, girls may have greater need for iron because of menstruation. Iron is widely distributed in foods, and sources include meats—especially liver—sardines, shrimp, oysters, green vegetables, dry beans, nuts, prunes, dates, and raisins. Because postpubescent boys grow at a faster rate and put on more muscle mass, their caloric requirements exceed those of girls.

Q. Shouldn't there be major changes in diet when a child reaches adolescence?

A. Not for the kind of balanced diet we talk about in this book. It provides for all the nutritional needs of both younger children and adolescents. There may, with adolescence, be changes in the way the body uses some nutrients. For example, protein. A younger child may not need all the protein available in the diet for the purpose of body building and so may use some of the protein simply as calories to be burned up for energy. An adolescent who is growing rapidly, however, may use all the protein for putting on additional body mass. But that doesn't mean that the diet, when it is sound and well balanced to begin with, has to be changed.

Q. Isn't it particularly harmful to restrict a child's eating at or around the time of puberty?

A. It's harmful, I think, at any age. When I say restrict, I mean restrict caloric intake to a level below that required to maintain ideal weight—in other words, to try to make a child lose weight rather than maintain weight. Because a child who eats the number of calories needed to maintain his ideal weight is actually consuming the number of calories correct for a child of his age. Restriction, I believe, is harmful to a child at any age, but is likely to be most harmful during adolescence because the body then is going through some of its most rapid changes. In fact, the only time growth is more rapid is during the first six months of life.

Q. How old does a child have to be to go on an adult kind of diet?

A. An adult kind of diet, if it is a sensible one, is not going to be any different from the kind of diet we advocate in this book. To be sure, unlike a child, an adult who is no longer growing cannot depend upon weight maintenance to grow into normal weight. However, even for the average over-weight adult, weight maintenance may be a good first goal. Many overweight people are in the process of gaining still more weight, and if they could stop further gains, that would be no small accomplishment. It might be easier for them to go on a weight-maintenance program and learn to eat prop-erly before rushing headlong into a more restrictive diet to lose weight. Once an adult is on an effective weight-mainte-nance diet, it can be much easier to reduce intake by, say, 100 calories a day, or perhaps a little more, and thus lose weight soundly and without intolerable-for-long discomfort.

Q. What do you think about having a child join a group such as Weight Watchers?

A. Organizations such as Weight Watchers and Overeaters Anonymous offer the advantage of group support, and the diets they recommend are well balanced. But before consider-ing having your child join a group, investigate the local chap-ter. There may be age requirements—and even if there aren't, the membership of the chapter may be so out of line with your child's age that he won't fit in and get the kind of group sup-port he needs, and so it may be of no benefit. In addition, groups that are geared mostly for dealing with adults may have no diet aimed at maintaining weight for a particular child. So while I believe their philosophy is good and their diets are well balanced, such groups may not be ideal for children. If you have an adolescent who might benefit from peer support, it may be possible for him or her to seek out other adolescents with weight problems who would like to try a weight-mainte-nance program once they know about it, and they might join with your child, getting together to discuss their plans, and how their diets are going, and give each other encourage-ment.

Q. *Since we can't serve diet food when we entertain guests, what can we do then?*

A. But you *can* serve diet food to guests. There is no reason food low in calories has to be unpalatable. And you can serve guests treats that you would not otherwise prepare. You may find, too, that your guests thoroughly enjoy low-calorie snacks —for example, fresh vegetables with dip, and with the dip made of low-fat yogurt rather than sour cream, or even of cottage cheese with some added spices.

Q. *Is it permissible to use wine in cooking?*

A. Yes. When you cook with wine, the alcohol evaporates and what is left is primarily flavoring, which will not add much in the way of calories.

Q. *Are any of the vast numbers of diet products on the market of value?*

A. There are a lot of products out on the market simply because desperate people are looking for simple solutions. There is no simple solution to obesity. To put it bluntly, there is nothing that can be taken out of a bottle or out of a can and put into your food or into your mouth that successfully can control weight for you over the long term.

Q. *My husband doesn't set a good example for our kids. He is fat, my two sons are, and my husband, always a meat-and-potatoes man, insists he always will be. What can I do about that in terms of the boys?*

A. In the process of helping your children grow slim, you don't, of course, want to suggest that Father is doing anything to their detriment. Nor do you want them bringing Father's weight up to him in any derogatory way. But your children don't have to eat exactly as their father does, and neither do you. To be sure, since meat and potatoes are perfectly normal foods to serve, your children can have them too—but not in the same quantities as your husband. And your husband, even though he may be a meat-and-potatoes man, would probably not find it objectionable if you used less fat and oil in preparing the meat and potatoes so they are lower in calo-ries—and he may even benefit from that. The question of what to do about a parent who doesn't want to cooperate in a diet depends partly on the age of the children. If you have younger children, I think setting goals for them can be achieved with the cooperation of that parent as long as he feels that nothing is going to be enforced on him. I don't think any father who is a meat-and-potatoes man would go so far as to insist that his children follow in his footsteps. Younger children, living a good portion of their lives seeing their father eating differently from the way they do, will wonder about it. The best one can hope to do is have both mother and father explain that Father has certain eating habits he finds difficult to break and they are not the best of all possible eating habits and he doesn't want the children to adopt them. With older children, there may be family battles. Especially as they suc-ceed in controlling their own weights, they may find their father's lack of control over his distasteful and may make quite an issue of it. I think that if Mother is the one sensible family member left in that situation, it becomes important for her to try to forestall a confrontation. If the dieting adolescent can be made to feel secure and good about himself, he may feel less of a need to point out the differences between himself and his father, and the more harmonious home environment will be better for the dieter and for everyone else in the family.

Q. We have tried your suggestions to help our child control his weight, but he is not at all interested, goes out of the house and eats all kinds of junk foods, and is still getting fatter and fatter. What can we do?

A. As long as you select foods and prepare them to provide sound, balanced meals which are not excessively high in cal-ories, you can have an environment that is not hostile to dieting and to maintaining healthy eating habits. No matter what your child does to keep himself from benefiting from this kind of environment, you should maintain it. If he succeeds in not gaining an additional pound or two in your home, it's a pound or two less than he would have put on if, after eating garbage on the outside, he came home to eat weight-adding meals. And sooner or later, when he becomes concerned enough about controlling his life and wanting to do something about his weight, he will have available a home environment that can help rather than hinder him.

Appendix A

GROWTH CHARTS

The following pages provide several sets of growth charts for boys and girls from ages 2 to 18 years.

For each child in the family, there is a chart "Stature for Age" along with another, "Weight for Age."

TO USE THE CHARTS

Take your child's present height and weight measurements with the child in minimal indoor clothing and without shoes.

Graph each measurement on the appropriate chart. To do this, first find the child's age on the horizontal line at the bottom of each chart.

Next, follow the vertical line extending upward from the age indication until it crosses the horizontal line representing the child's stature (height) or weight.

Finally, where the two lines intersect on each chart, pencil a cross mark.

You now know in which percentiles* the child's height and weight fall.

When, for example, a cross mark is on the 95th-percentile line of weight for age, it means that only 5 children among

---

* *The percentiles for these charts were established by the U.S. National Center for Health Statistics in collaboration with the Centers for Disease Control and are based on data from national probability samples representative of boys and girls in the general population.*

100 of the same age and sex have weights greater than your child's.

Is the child overweight? He may well be, as indicated in Chapter 2, if he is in a much higher percentile for weight than for height.

You can also use the charts to find the child's *ideal* weight —or the age at which his or her present weight will become ideal if it is maintained. The ideal occurs when both height and weight fall on the same percentile curve.

Also provided in the following pages are growth charts with percentiles for girls and boys from birth to 36 months of age. They are based on data from the Fels Research Institute, Yellow Springs, Ohio. You can use them in the same way to determine whether stature and weight percentiles match or come close to matching or whether the child's weight percentile is significantly higher than the stature percentile, indicating likely overweight.

AN ADDITIONAL AID

Still another type of chart—"Weight for Stature"—is provided as an additional means of determining whether a child is overweight.

Here, you plot weight against height.

To do so, simply find the child's height in inches on the horizontal line at the bottom of the chart. Then follow the vertical line extending upward from the height indication until it crosses the horizontal line representing the child's weight.

Where the two lines intersect, pencil a cross mark.

If the mark is above the 95th-percentile curve, the child is clearly obese. If the mark is above the 90th but below the 95th percentile, the child is somewhat overweight. If the mark is below the 90th percentile, the decision as to whether there is a weight problem depends on how mother and/or child feel about the child's appearance.

The chart can be helpful, too, when it is used over a period of years and the latest measurements of height and weight are plotted from time to time—perhaps every 6 months, or even more frequently.

It can show, from one period to the next, whether the child's development is continuing in the same percentile or the weight percentile is, undesirably, increasing, indicating a weight problem.

BOYS FROM 2 TO 18 YEARS
STATURE FOR AGE

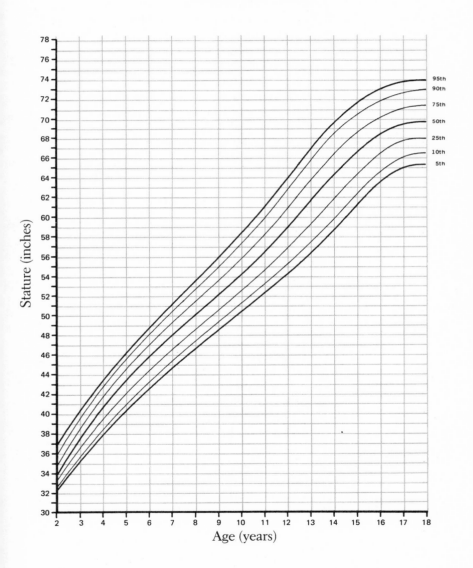

BOYS FROM 2 TO 18 YEARS

WEIGHT FOR AGE

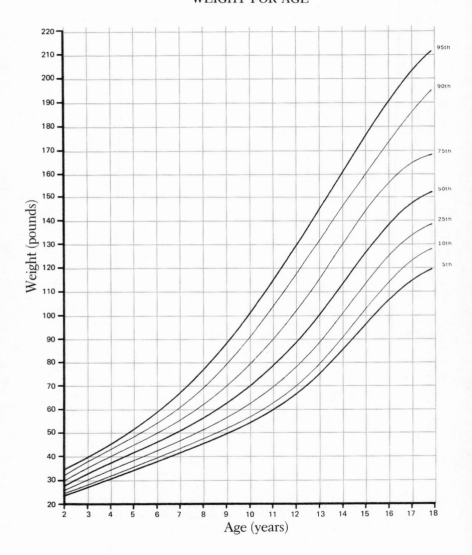

PREPUBERTAL BOYS FROM 2 TO 11½ YEARS
WEIGHT FOR STATURE

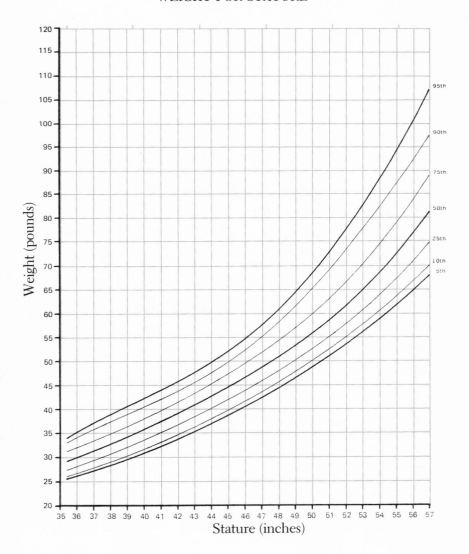

95th
90th
75th
50th
25th
10th
5th

Weight (pounds)

Stature (inches)

GIRLS FROM 2 TO 18 YEARS

STATURE FOR AGE

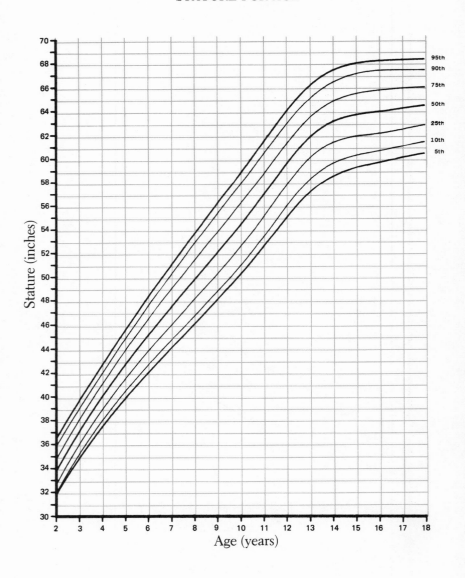

GIRLS FROM 2 TO 18 YEARS

WEIGHT FOR AGE

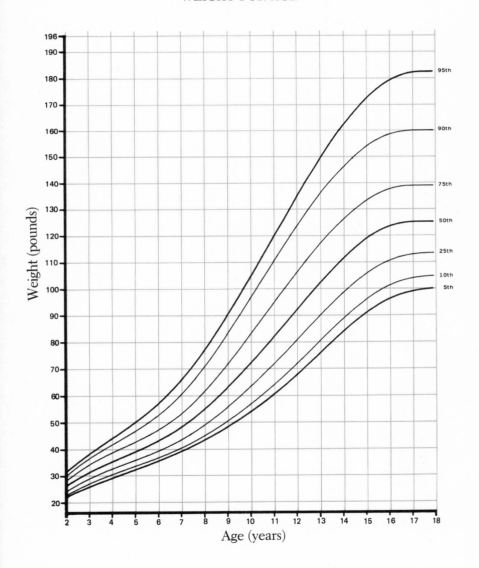

PREPUBERTAL GIRLS FROM 2 TO 10 YEARS
WEIGHT FOR STATURE

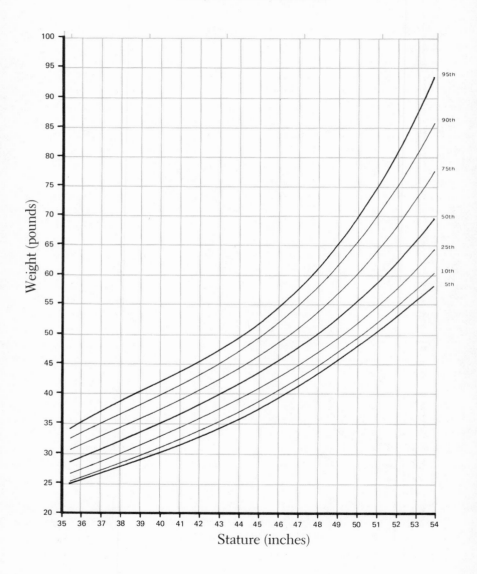

BOYS FROM BIRTH TO 36 MONTHS

WEIGHT FOR AGE

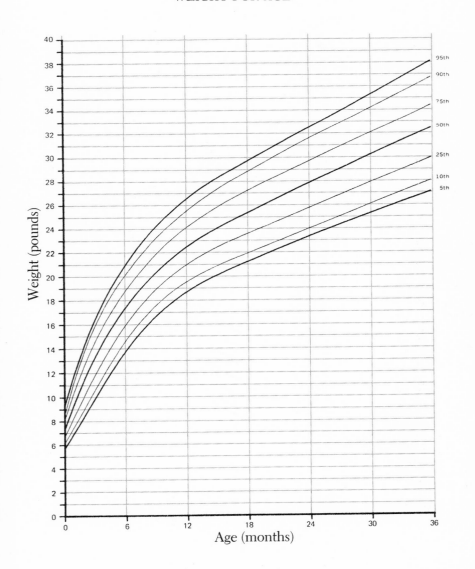

BOYS FROM BIRTH TO 36 MONTHS
LENGTH FOR AGE

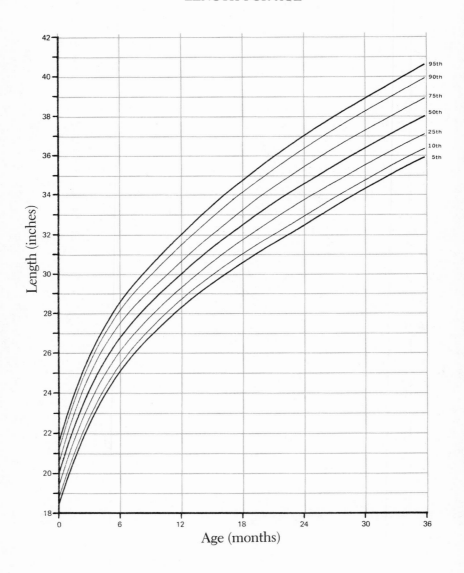

BOYS FROM BIRTH TO 36 MONTHS

WEIGHT FOR LENGTH

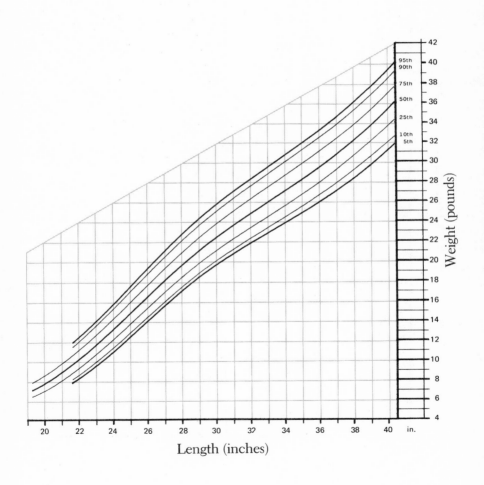

95th
90th
75th
50th
25th
10th
5th

Weight (pounds)

Length (inches)

GIRLS FROM BIRTH TO 36 MONTHS
LENGTH FOR AGE

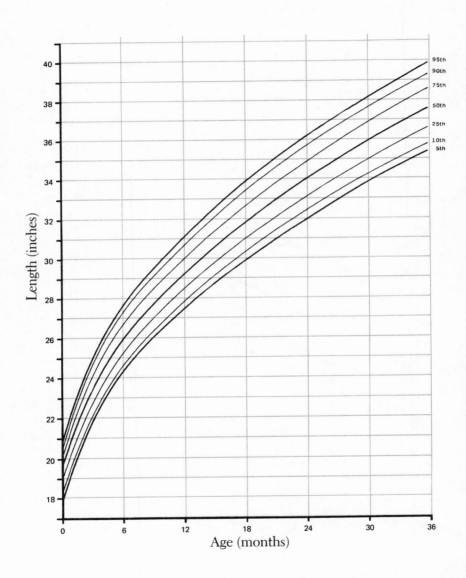

GIRLS FROM BIRTH TO 36 MONTHS

WEIGHT FOR AGE

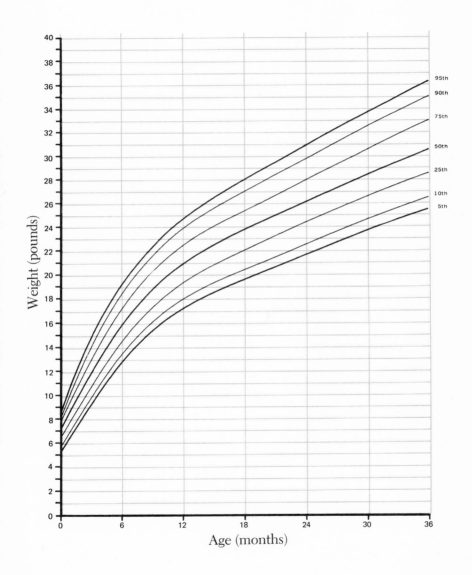

GIRLS FROM BIRTH TO 36 MONTHS
WEIGHT FOR LENGTH

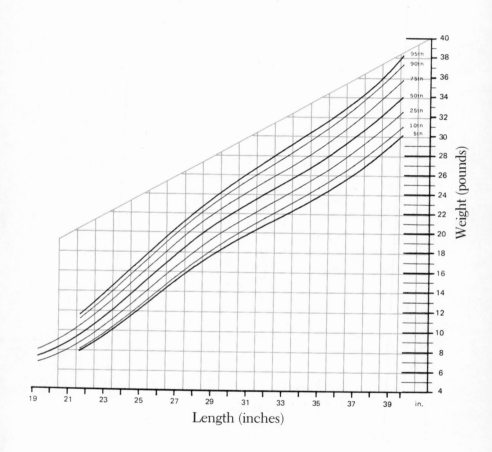

Appendix B

PARENT MID-STATURE CHART

Parental midpoint in inches

Age (years)	63 3/8	64 3/16	65	65 3/4	66 1/2	67 5/16	68 1/8	68 7/8	69 11/16	70
			Approximate predicted height (inches) for age							
GIRLS 15	61 3/8	62 1/16	62 5/8	63 1/4	63 13/16	64 3/8	65	65 1/2	66	66 5/16
16	61 7/16	62 1/16	62 11/16	63 5/16	63 15/16	64 9/16	65 1/4	65 7/8	66 1/2	66 13/16
17	61 1/2	62 3/16	62 7/8	63 9/16	64 1/4	64 15/16	65 5/8	66 5/16	67	67 5/16
18	61 1/2	62 3/16	62 15/16	63 5/8	64 3/8	65 1/16	65 13/16	66 1/2	67 1/4	67 5/8
BOYS 15		65 1/4	65 13/16	66 3/8	66 15/16	67 1/2	68 1/16	68 5/8	69 3/16	69 7/16
16		66 11/16	67 5/16	67 15/16	68 9/16	69 3/16	69 13/16	70 7/16	71 1/16	71 5/16
17		67 1/4	67 15/16	68 5/8	69 3/8	70 1/16	70 3/4	71 7/16	72 1/8	72 9/16
18		67 1/2	68 1/4	69 1/16	69 13/16	70 9/16	71 3/8	72 1/8	72 7/8	73 5/16

Adapted from Fels Parent-Specific Standards for Height. Adjusted by extrapolation.

This is an alternative means of predicting height at a given age and also can be used to predict final height. Final height usually occurs at about 18 years of age, but may occur earlier with early completion of sexual maturation.

To find your predicted height for a given age, find your parental midpoint by adding both parents' heights in inches and dividing by 2. Your predicted height appears in your parental midpoint column across from your age.

Appendix C

CALORIC REQUIREMENTS

AVERAGE DAILY CALORIC REQUIREMENTS BY WEIGHT AT VARIOUS AGES

AGE (YEARS)	CALORIES/POUND
Infancy	50
1–3	45
4–6	41
7–9	36
10–12	32
13–15	27
15+	23
Adult	18

AVERAGE DAILY CALORIC REQUIREMENTS BY AGE

AGE (YEARS)	BOYS	GIRLS
1–2	1,100	1,100
2–3	1,300	1,300
3–4	1,400	1,400
4–6	1,600	1,600
6–8	2,000	2,000
8–10	2,200	2,200
10–12	2,500	2,300
12–14	2,700	2,300
14–18	3,000	2,300
18–22	2,800	2,000

Appendix D

TABLE OF FOOD VALUES*

The following table shows the approximate caloric values of foods and the amounts of protein, fat, and carbohydrate in usual portions.

Volume measurements are indicated as tsp (teaspoon), tbsp (tablespoon), or fractions of a cup (8 ounces), while weight measurements are given in ounces. The amounts of protein, fat, and carbohydrate per portion are noted in grams (100 grams equal approximately 3½ ounces) so that foods may be readily compared with each other and with the exchange lists in Chapter 8.

All portions listed are weighed or measured after cooking except for fruits, many dairy foods, and some vegetables which are eaten raw. Cooked-vegetable portions are boiled or steamed.

Differences in cooking method can significantly alter caloric content: frying adds fat, whereas broiling removes fat and water.

Meat portions are lean cuts with excess fat removed. Gourmet meat cuts which are well marbled with fat may have significantly more calories and fat even if trimmed.

---

* Derived from The Handbook of the Nutritional Contents of Foods prepared for the U.S. Department of Agriculture by Bernice K. Watt and Annabel L. Merrill, published by Dover Publications, 1975.

FOOD	PORTION	CAL-ORIES	PROTEIN (GRAMS)	FAT (GRAMS)	CARBO-HYDRATE (GRAMS)
Almonds	½ cup (2½ oz.)	425	13.2	38.4	13.8
Apple	small, 2½″ dia. 3.5 oz.	60	.2	.7	14.8
Applesauce, unsweetened	½ cup	50	.2	.2	13.1
Apricots, dried	½ cup, halves	200	3.8	.4	51
Apricots, fresh	3 medium	50	1.0	.2	12.8
Bacon	2 slices (½ oz., cooked)	100	5.0	8.5	.5
Banana	1 med. (6″)	90	1.2	.2	23.5
Beans, baked	½ cup	150	7.9	.6	28.8
Beans, green or wax	½ cup	15	1.0	.1	3.0
Beans, lima	½ cup, cooked	75	5.1	.3	13.4
Beef, corned	2 oz.	210	13.0	17.2	0
Beef, hamburger	4 oz., broiled	325	27.4	23.0	0
Beef, roast	4 oz., roasted	360	28.2	26.5	0
Beef, roast	4 oz., broiled	300	32.4	17.5	0
Beef, steak, lean, fat-trimmed	4 oz., broiled	300	32.4	17.5	0
Beets	½ cup	30	1.1	.1	7.2
Biscuit	1, 2½″ dia.	125	2.5	5.7	15.5
Blackberries	½ cup	40	.8	.6	8.9
Blueberries	½ cup	40	.7	.3	10.4
Bologna, all-meat	2 oz.	160	7.5	12.9	2.1
Bran, raisin	½ cup	80	2.0	.7	18.7
Bran flakes, 40% bran	½ cup	55	1.9	.3	14.8
Bread, French	3 × 3½″ oval, ½″ slice	55	1.7	.6	10.5
Bread, Italian	3 × 3½″ oval, ½″ slice	50	1.6	.1	10.2
Bread, raisin	1 slice	80	2.0	.9	16.4
Bread, rye or pumpernickel	1 slice	60	2.2	.3	12.9
Bread, white	1 slice	65	2.1	.8	12.2
Bread, whole-wheat	1 slice	55	2.4	.7	10.8

FOOD	PORTION	CAL-ORIES	PROTEIN (GRAMS)	FAT (GRAMS)	CARBO-HYDRATE (GRAMS)
Broccoli	½ cup	20	2.6	.3	3.8
Brussels sprouts	½ cup	25	2.9	.3	4.4
Butter	1 pat (½ tbsp)	50	trace	5.6	trace
Cabbage	½ cup	20	1.1	.2	4.3
Cake, angel-food	⅟₁₂, 8″ dia.	110	2.9	.1	24.6
Cake, pound	¾″ slice	130	1.6	8.1	12.9
Cantaloupe	½, 5″ dia.	40	.9	.1	10.0
Carrots, cooked	½ cup	20	.5	.1	4.6
Carrots, raw	1, 5½″	20	.5	.1	4.6
Cashew nuts	1 oz.	160	4.9	13.0	8.3
Cauliflower	½ cup	15	1.6	.1	2.8
Celery	1 large stalk (½ cup)	10	.5	.1	2.3
Cheese, American	1-oz. slice	100	6.6	8.5	.5
Cheese, Cheddar	1 oz.	110	7.1	9.1	.6
Cheese, cottage, low-fat	½ cup	90	16.0	1	4.0
Cheese, cream	1 tbsp	60	1.3	6.0	.3
Cheese, Swiss	1 oz.	100	7.8	7.9	.5
Cherries	½ cup	35	.7	.2	8.6
Chicken	4 oz. roasted, no skin	200	34.9	5.7	0
Cod	4 oz., broiled	190	32.3	6.0	0
Cookies, butter	1	40	.5	1.5	6.2
Cookies, choc-olate-chip	1	50	.6	2.2	7.4
Cookies, fig bar	1	60	.7	.9	12.6
Cookies, oatmeal with raisins	1	55	.8	1.9	9.0
Cookies, sand-wich creme	1	50	.5	2.3	7.0
Cookies, vanilla wafer	1	20	.2	.7	3.2
Corn	½ cup	70	2.7	.8	15.9
Corn on cob	5″	80	2.9	.9	18.5
Cornflakes	½ cup	50	1.0	.1	11.0
Crab	4 oz. steamed	105	19.6	2.2	.6
Crackers, graham	3½″ square	25	.5	.6	4.8

149

FOOD	PORTION	CAL-ORIES	PROTEIN (GRAMS)	FAT (GRAMS)	CARBO-HYDRATE (GRAMS)
Crackers, saltine	2" square	20	.4	.6	3.3
Cranberries	½ cup	25	.2	.4	5.9
Cranberry sauce	2 tbsp	70	.1	.1	18.8
Cucumber	1, 7"	25	1.5	.2	5.7
Egg	1, raw or boiled	80	6.3	5.8	.4
Eggplant	3½ oz.	25	1.2	.2	5.6
Farina	½ cup, cooked	50	1.5	.1	10.3
Flounder	4 oz., baked	230	34.0	9.3	0
Frankfurter	1, 1½ oz.	125	5.6	10.8	1.1
Fruit cocktail	½ cup	90	.5	.1	23.3
Grapefruit	½, 4" dia.	75	1.0	.2	18.0
Grapefruit juice, un-sweetened	8 oz.	90	1.3	.4	21.1
Grape juice	8 oz.	170	.5	.1	42.8
Grapes	½ cup	50	1.0	.8	12.0
Halibut	4 oz., broiled	195	28.6	7.9	0
Ice cream	1 scoop (½ cup)	145	3.4	8.0	15.6
Ice milk	1 scoop (½ cup)	85	2.7	2.85	12.5
Jams, jellies	1 tbsp	50	.1	trace	12.9
Lamb, roast leg	4 oz.	315	28.7	21.4	0
Lamb chop, rib	4 oz. broiled	460	22.8	40.4	0
Lettuce	2 large or 4 small leaves	7	.6	.1	1.8
Liver, beef	4 oz., fried	260	29.9	12.0	6.0
Liver, chicken	4 oz., simmered	190	30.0	5.0	3.5
Lobster	4 oz., boiled	105	21.2	1.7	.3
Macaroni	½ cup, cooked	100	3.1	.4	20.7
Margarine	1 pat (½ tbsp)	50	trace	5.6	trace
Mayonnaise	1 tbsp	90	.1	10.0	.3
Milk, skim	1 cup (8 oz.)	85	8.5	.2	12.0
Milk, 2%	1 cup (8 oz.)	120	8.0	5.0	11.0
Milk, whole	1 cup (8 oz.)	165	8.8	8.8	12.3
Muffin: blueberry, corn, English	1	130	3.4	4.4	19.0
Mushrooms	½ cup, raw	10	.9	.1	1.4
Noodles	½ cup, cooked	100	3.3	1.2	18.7

FOOD	PORTION	CAL-ORIES	PROTEIN (GRAMS)	FAT (GRAMS)	CARBO-HYDRATE (GRAMS)
Oatmeal	½ cup, cooked	75	2.7	1.4	13.2
Olives, green	5 (1 oz.)	35	.4	3.6	.4
Onions	½ cup, boiled	40	1.7	.1	9.0
Onions	1 oz., raw	10	.4	trace	2.5
Orange	1 medium (3″)	70	1.4	.3	17.4
Orange juice	1 cup (8 oz.)	120	2.0	.5	28.0
Pancake	1, 4″ dia.	60	1.8	1.8	8.9
Peach, fresh	1 med.	50	.8	.1	12.8
Peanut butter	2 tbsp	190	8.0	17.0	6.0
Peanuts, roasted	¼ cup	200	9.0	16.7	7.1
Pear	1 med.	95	1.1	.6	23.8
Peas	½ cup	70	5.4	.4	12.1
Pecans	¼ cup	190	2.5	19.5	4.0
Pepper, green, sweet	1 med.	15	.8	.1	3.3
Pickle, dill or sour	1, 4″ long	15	.8	.3	3.1
Pie, apple	⅛, 9″	290	2.5	12.6	43.2
Pie, lemon meringue	⅛, 9″	265	3.8	10.6	39.2
Pie, pumpkin	⅛, 9″	230	4.4	12.2	26.7
Pineapple	1 cup	75	.6	.3	19.8
Pineapple juice	1 cup	120	.9	.2	29.5
Pizza	1 slice	240	14.0	9.0	25.0
Plum	1, 2″ dia.	30	.2	trace	8.1
Popcorn, plain	1 cup	65	2.1	.8	12.9
Pork, ham	4 oz. lean	390	27.4	30.5	0
Pork, loin chop	4 oz. broiled	445	28.0	35.9	0
Potato	1 med., boiled or baked	100	2.8	.1	22.5
Potato	10 French-fried	200	3.1	9.6	26.3
Potato chips	1 oz. (15 chips)	160	1.5	11.3	14.2
Pretzels	1 oz.	110	2.8	1.3	21.5
Prune	1 uncooked	20	.2	trace	5.3
Raisins	2 tbsp	60	.6	trace	15.4
Raspberries black	½ cup	55	1.1	1.1	11.8
Raspberries, red	½ cup	40	.8	.4	9.5
Rice	½ cup, boiled	100	2.0	.1	24.2
Salad dressing, low-fat French	1 tsp	11	trace	1.0	1.0
Salad dressing, low-fat Italian	1 tsp	3	trace	.3	.2

FOOD	PORTION	CAL-ORIES	PROTEIN (GRAMS)	FAT (GRAMS)	CARBO-HYDRATE (GRAMS)
Salmon	4 oz., broiled or baked	205	30.6	8.4	0
Sardines	4 oz., drained	230	27.2	12.6	1.9
Sauerkraut	½ cup	20	1.0	.2	4.0
Scallops	4 oz., steamed	125	26.3	1.6	1.4
Shrimp	4 oz., boiled or steamed	130	27.4	1.2	.8
Spaghetti	½ cup, cooked	110	3.4	.4	23.0
Spinach	½ cup	25	3.0	.3	3.6
Squash, summer	½ cup	15	.9	.1	3.1
Squash, winter	½ cup	45	1.5	.1	11.2
Strawberries, fresh	½ cup	25	.5	.4	6.1
Sugar: beet, cane, brown	1 tsp	18	0	0	4.7
Sweet potato	1 med., baked	200	2.9	.7	45.5
Tangerine	1 med., 2½"	35	.6	.2	8.8
Tomato	1 med., 2½"	30	1.5	.3	6.4
Tomato juice	1 cup	50	2.4	.3	11.3
Tuna	3½ oz., drained	200	28.8	8.2	0
Turkey	4 oz., roasted, no skin	300	30.6	18.6	0
Turnips	½ cup	30	1.0	.3	8.6
Veal	4 oz., broiled	265	31.6	14.5	0
Walnuts	2 tbsp.	100	2.3	9.8	2.4
Watermelon	½ slice, ½"	45	.9	.3	11.1
Wheat, shredded, cereal	1 2" square	80	2.2	.5	8.1
Wheat, puffed	½ cup	75	3.0	.3	15.7
Yogurt	1 cup, low-fat, fruit	260	10.0	3.0	49.0
Yogurt	1 cup, low-fat, plain	150	12.0	4.0	17.0
Zucchini	½ cup, boiled	25	1.1	.2	5.9

Index

hydrogenation, 44
hypertension, 77
hypoglycemia, 25, 27, 72
hypothyroidism, 36, 96

ice skating, 86
ideal weight, 10, 13, 18–20, 119, 132
  growing into, 12, 13
  for late adolescence, 19–20
  reducing and, 18–19
illnesses:
  dieting and, 120–21
  obesity and, 30–31, 124
  stress as cause of, 78
infections, 9, 45
insomnia, 94, 95
insulin, 25, 47
International Units, 44
intertrigo, 32
intestinal disturbances, 78
intestines, 44, 45
iodine, 47
iron, 45, 47, 126
irritability, 31, 46, 94, 96
isoleucine, 39

jogging, 80, 87
Johns Hopkins University,
  infant study of, 103
junk foods, 71–72
  eaten during illness, 120
  weight gain and, 119–20

ketone bodies, 26–27, 28
ketosis, 26–29
  side effects of, 27
kidneys, 27, 39, 78
kidney stones, 46

lactose, 41
lanugo, 114
learning interferences, 9
leucine, 39
lips, 46
liquid protein diets, 25–26
  side effects of, 26
liver, 27, 39
log, diet, 49–50, 71, 120
loneliness, as cause of
  overeating, 50
low blood sugar, 25, 27, 72

lungs, 27
lymphatic system, 27
lysine, 39

macronutrients, 47
magnesium, 47
malnourishment:
  harmful effects of, 9
  see also anorexia nervosa
maltose, 41
manganese, 47–48
Mayer, Jean, 80
Mayo Clinic, 23
"Mayo" diet, 23
meats:
  diet exchanges for, 66
  fats in, 43, 44
  minerals in, 47–48, 126
  overemphasis of, 40–41
  preparation of, 58
  proteins in, 39–41
Medical Letter, 29, 93, 94
menstruation, 126
  anorexia nervosa and, 114
mental achievement, exercise
  and, 77
Merrill, Annabel L., 147*n*
methionine, 39
micrograms, 44
micronutrients, 47
milk and milk products, *see*
  dairy products
milligrams, 44
minerals, 39, 42, 46–48
molybdenum, 48
mothers:
  as diet enforcers, 19
  as molders of baby's appetite,
    103
  rejection of obese children by,
    33
mouth, 46
muscles, 39, 42, 47, 48, 110, 125
musculoskeletal system, 31

nasal passages, 45
National Basketball Association,
  86
National Basketball Players
  Association, 85–86
nausea, 46, 94, 96
nerves, 45, 48

stress, 9
  exercise and, 78–79
  illnesses caused by, 78
  overeating due to, 22
strokes, 30
sucrose, 41
sugar, refined, 24–25, 31, 42, 43
sugars, 41
Surgeon General's Report,
  U.S., 79
swallowing mechanism, 105–6,
  110
swayback, 32
swimming, 80, 86

taste, 36
teeth, 46
tennis, 86, 87
tension, 78, 79
thiamine (B_1), 41, 45, 46
thighs, fat accumulation on, 31–
  32
threonine, 39
thyroid compounds, 96
thyroid gland, 35, 36, 96
thyroid hormones, 36
tongue, 46
tooth decay, 25, 46
trace elements, 41, 47
treats, 72–73, 121–22
  relatives and, 122–23
tremors, 95
triglycerides, 36
tryptophan, 39, 44
Tutko, Thomas, 83–84

underweight, misconceptions
  about, 108–9
unsaturated fats, 44
urinalysis, 36
urine, 27

valine, 39
vegetable oils, 44
vegetables, 52, 95
  children and, 122–23
  diet exchanges for, 63, 65
  minerals in, 47–48, 126
  preparation of, 58, 124

proteins in, 39–40
starches in, 41–42
vitamins in, 46
vitamin A, 43, 45, 46
vitamin B complex, 41, 44, 45,
  46
vitamin C, 41, 42, 45, 46
vitamin D, 43, 44, 45, 46
vitamin E, 43, 45, 46
vitamin K, 43, 44, 45, 46
vitamins, 38, 39, 41, 42, 43, 44–
  46
  classification of, 45
  conditions caused by lack of,
    46
  function of, 44–45

walking, overweight and, 30–31
Wall Street Journal, The, 84–85
water:
  in baby food, 110
  diuretics and, 95–96, 114
  weight loss and, 23, 29, 75
"water pills," 95–96, 114
Watt, Bernice K., 147n
weight:
  exercise and, 79–81
  ideal, *see* ideal weight
  myths and misconceptions
    about, 103, 108–9
  recording of, 75
  thyroid hormones and, 36
weight charts, 13–18, 19–20,
  131–44
weight-control plan:
  aspects of, 9–10
  goal of, 13
  see also zero-weight-gain plan
Weight Watchers, 127
Wellington, Duke of (Arthur
  Wellesley), 28
wines, 128
*Winning Is Everything—and
  Other American Myths*
  (Tutko and Bruns), 83–84

YMCAs, 84–86
Youth Basketball Association
  (YBA), 84–86

159